Are You an Attorney or Advisor?

The professional edition of this book, ***Medicaid Planning: From A to Z***, contains:

- 538 full-size (8.5" x 11") pages
- 500+ footnotes (every citation—law, rule, regulation, and case reference— is cited in full; a HUGE timesaver that vastly speeds up your research: worth the cost of the manual alone!)
- Additional in-depth discussions aimed at the attorney/advisor
- Two additional chapters on Medicaid Planning and Attorney Professional Ethics (39 pages—used with a two-hour ethics CLE course)
- Sample legal forms, including: Durable Power of Attorney; Will with Elective Share Trust; Promissory Note; Ladybird Deed; Deed of Small Percentage Interest (ready to be incorporated into your legal forms, for all your Medicaid clients)
- 138 pages of the most-used Medicaid statutes and regulations so they are at your fingertips
- A completed Medicaid application as an example to guide you
- Entire book re-written specifically for the attorney/advisor

- For more information, visit:

www.MedicaidSecrets.com

Special Editions/Bulk Purchases

This book is available for special discounts for bulk purchases for sales promotions or premiums. Special editions, including personalized covers, excerpts of existing books, and corporate imprints, can be created in large quantities for special needs. For more information, email Murphy & Berglund, PLLC at info@murphyberglund.com.

HOW TO PROTECT YOUR FAMILY'S ASSETS FROM DEVASTATING NURSING HOME COSTS

Medicaid Secrets

2025 Edition

Jodi E. Murphy, Attorney

Michelle A. Berglund-Harper, Attorney

This publication is designed to provide accurate and authoritative information in regard to the subject matter covered. It is sold with the understanding that the publisher is not engaged in rendering legal, accounting, or other professional service. If legal advice or other expert assistance is required, the services of a competent professional should be sought.

—From a *Declaration of Principles* jointly adopted by a committee of the American Bar Association and a committee of publishers and associations

Published by:

Murphy & Berglund, PLLC

1101 Douglas Avenue Suite 1006

Altamonte Springs, FL 32714

407-865-9553

info@murphyberglund.com

Library of Congress Control Number: 2019919777

For additional copies: www.MedicaidSecrets.com

ABOUT THE AUTHOR

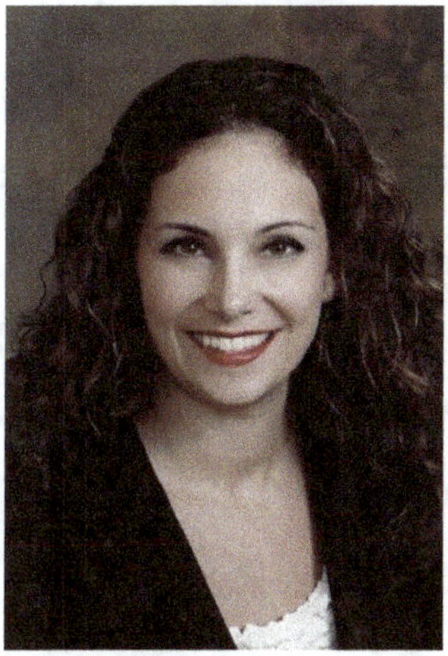

Jodi E. Murphy

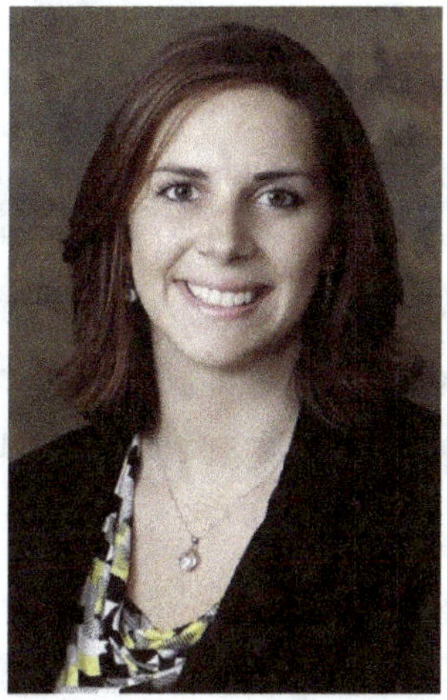

Michelle A. Berglund-Harper

The law firm of Murphy & Berglund, PLLC was established with the objective of providing estate planning for all Florida residents, from basic will planning to complex trust planning. The firm focuses on protecting every branch of a client's family tree through estate planning with a comprehensive plan that takes into account all of a family's ever-changing needs.

Attorney Jodi Murphy is the head of the benefits planning department of Murphy & Berglund, PLLC. Her practice areas include trust and estate planning, Medicaid planning and Veterans Benefits planning. Prior to establishing her own firm in 2006, Jodi Murphy was a litigation and family law associate with Baker & Hostetler, LLP (Orlando, FL).

Attorney Michelle A. Berglund-Harper is the head of the litigation department at Murphy & Berglund, PLLC. Her practice areas include Estate Planning, Elder law, Medicaid and VA Benefits Planning, Probate planning and administration, Trust Administration, Guardianship law, and Real Estate. Prior to partnering with Attorney Jodi Murphy in 2011, Michelle Berglund-Harper ran her own firm (Orlando, FL) which focused primarily on family law, and representing victims of domestic violence.

Attorneys Murphy & Berglund-Harper take pride in assisting clients to care for loved ones through thoughtful, intentional planning and are active in their communities, speaking as a panelist and hosting seminars regularly.

With over 35 years of combined legal experience, the attorneys have counseled many clients and attorneys in *Medicaid and VA planning*. In 2013, the attorneys began to co-author this book with hopes of reaching a national audience. The attorneys also co-author a book Medicaid Planning from A-Z which is a comprehensive guide for professionals who are looking to branch out into new practice areas.

To invite one of the attorneys to speak at your next seminar, please contact info@murphyberglund.com.

TABLE OF CONTENTS

Chapter 1

INTRODUCTION

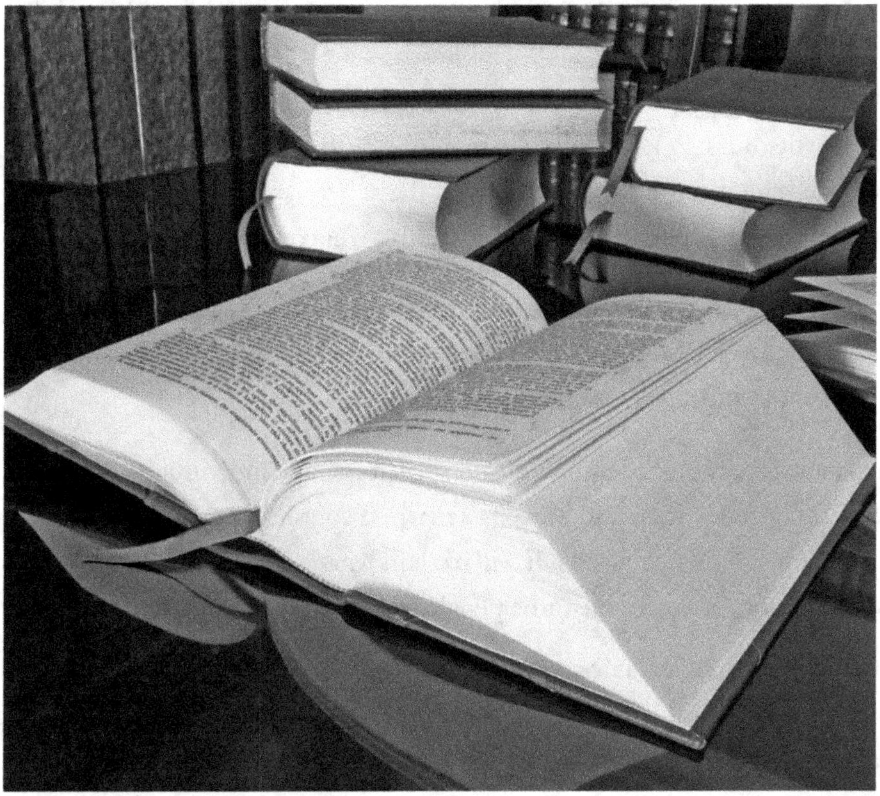

You are reading this book because you already know the cold, hard facts: nursing homes are expensive, and without careful planning, a stay in one can easily bankrupt all but the most affluent families. Considering that the average cost of a nursing home in the U.S. exceeds $9,800 a month, with costs increasing every year you're looking at a bill of over $588,000 for your family member with Alzheimer's disease, whose nursing home stay typically is five years or more.

What most people don't realize is that, as a general rule, the government will only pay the nursing home bill if your cash is below $2,000. Medicare will only cover you for a maximum of 100 days, if they cover you at all; Social Security won't cover these bills, either. Only Medicaid will cover you— if you qualify!

This book will explain in plain English what the rules are and how you can qualify for Medicaid coverage of your nursing home bills yet still protect your home and life savings.

This book covers the federal Medicaid rules for single individuals (divorced, widowed, or never married) as well as married couples. It will discuss both the income limits and asset limits. It will explain what you can do—to protect your assets and not get in trouble or be penalized—and what you cannot do.

Without proper legal advice, you will undoubtedly be told that you must spend down your assets until you have reduced your life savings to the point that you qualify for Medicaid coverage of your nursing home bills. Unfortunately, this leaves you without the cash to pay for items and "extras" not paid for by the Medicaid program. What if your family wants to visit you and you'd like to pay their way? What if you want some new clothes? A large-screen TV? Remote headphones so you can hear your TV better? Specialized or alternative medical treatments not covered by Medicaid? Without some source of private funds, you will be at the mercy of the Medicaid program. If they don't pay for it, you're simply out of luck.

Also, most people with children would prefer to be able to pass on at least part of their life savings—and hopefully the family home or farm—to their children.

And many people without children would still prefer to give their assets either to other family members- siblings, nieces, nephews- or to their church, synagogue or other charitable or educational institution, than to use up every dime of their life savings paying for their last years in a nursing home.

It is important to note that, while all the advice given in this book is completely legal, some techniques may not work in all states. The reason for this is that the Medicaid system, while based on federal law, allows each state to select certain optional rules. Accordingly, the Medicaid rules reflect a crazy patchwork quilt of federal rules, regulations, and cases, and state statutes, regulations, and case law. As if that weren't bad enough, what may be approved in one county—or even by one caseworker within a single county—may not fly in a different county or by a different caseworker.

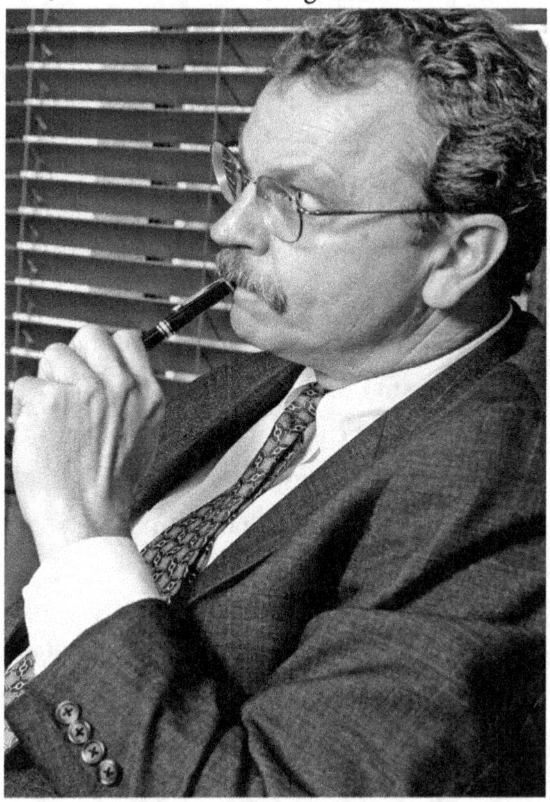

Sometimes the decisions of the caseworker will be wrong, and you will need to appeal to a higher level supervisor, or even request a mini-trial known as a "Fair Hearing." The point is that you cannot simply take the information here at face value without checking with a local elder law attorney who is familiar with your state's Medicaid rules—and, just as importantly, the unwritten policy and procedures used by the caseworker in your local county. However, after reading this book you will know what to ask the attorney and you will have some idea what is in store for your family.

How to Use This Book

As you can see from the introduction, the Medicaid system is extremely complex. Your facts and circumstances will differ from those of everyone else in the following ways:

- Age, health, and life expectancy of the potential Medicaid applicant
- Marital status of the applicant
- If married, the age, health, and life expectancy of the potential Medicaid applicant's spouse
- Type of assets held in the name of the applicant (and spouse, if any)
    - Is there a home? A family farm?
    - Family business?
    - IRAs or other retirement accounts?
- Total amount of assets held in the name of the applicant (and spouse, if any)
- Total amount of income, including pensions and Social Security, of the applicant (and spouse, if any)
- Number of children in the applicant's family
- Family dynamics
- Location of various family members
- Other unique factors

Every example given in this book may not apply to your particular situation. As stated above, the laws of your state may not permit a specific technique discussed in the book. In addition, the laws, rules, and regulations may have changed in your state since the time this was written. The Affordable Care Act's Medicaid expansion expanded Medicaid coverage to nearly all adults with incomes up to 138% of the Federal Poverty Level and provided states with an enhanced federal matching rate for their expansion populations. To date, 41 states (including DC) have adopted the Medicaid expansion and 10 states have not. Thus, we are in a transition period, further complicating matters. For a complete list of states that have adopted the expansion act visit https://www.kff.org/affordable-care-act/issue-brief/status-of-state-medicaid-expansion-decisions-interactive-map/.

As a result, the only sure way to know what will work, and what is best for your particular situation, is to consult an elder law attorney (see *How to Find the Right Kind of Attorney*, in the Appendix). In other words, **do not attempt to put any of the ideas in this book into place without the assistance of a specialist elder law attorney! To do otherwise is to risk your life savings.**

> **While this book won't replace the need to consult with an experienced elder law attorney, it will tell you what you need to know to make sure you are getting good advice. In addition, by showing up to your appointment with your lawyer armed with a list of relevant questions and a good understanding of the Medicaid rules, you'll not only save time, but you'll most likely reduce your legal bill, too.**

Thus, the best way to use this book is as an **Idea Book**. It can stimulate your thinking and arm you with lots of great ideas and concepts to bring to your attorney. It will educate you on both the basic concepts of the Medicaid system as it applies to anyone living in a nursing home as well as more advanced asset protection techniques. And, most importantly, it can keep you from making mistakes. Once you become aware of the planning possibilities available to you, hopefully, you will steer clear of making the kinds of transfers or blunders that can get you in trouble down the road!

As you read through the book, check off or highlight any ideas that you think may apply to your particular situation. Discuss them with your family members and finally bring them to the attention of your attorney. Your attorney can then evaluate them in light of your state's laws as well as the financial and health status of the family member who is planning on applying for Medicaid coverage.

Is It legal?

Have no fears—every technique and option discussed in this book is 100% legal! As attorneys with over 20 years of experience, we would never suggest any planning technique or option that is not legal. For example, simply "hiding" money is not an option: to do so and not report the asset on a Medicaid application is clearly a fraud against the state and federal governments, with severe legal consequences. There are ample ways to achieve your goals using completely legal methods. Don't risk going to jail or incurring huge fines and penalties by doing anything illegal!

Is It Ethical?

Some people simply do not like the fact that there are attorneys who specialize in advising clients how to save their money and qualify for Medicaid coverage sooner. Their theory is that Medicaid is a "welfare" program for the poor, broke, and destitute, and was not designed as a way for middle class parents to pass their money on to their children at taxpayer expense.

My answer to this is as follows:

> John Jones lives next door to Sam Smith. Both of these fine fellows are age 75 and have about $100,000 in the bank and a home that is paid off. John has a friend named Joe who lives across town in an apartment, who used to have some savings but who squandered it on drink and gambling.
>
> John has a heart attack and is rushed to the hospital. Thank goodness he survives, but the operation costs $80,000. Lucky for him he's covered by Medicare, so he arrives home with his life savings intact. Upon his death, his $100,000 and his home pass to his children, under his will.
>
> Meanwhile, Sam has a stroke and has to be moved to a nursing home. Since the nursing home costs $8,000 a month, Sam's life savings are gone in about a year. At that point, Sam qualifies for Medicaid, which pays his nursing home bills. He continues to reside in the nursing home

> for two more years, and upon his death the state has spent another $200,000 on his care. Under federal law, the state must be repaid at Sam's death, and since the only asset in his name is his house, it has to be sold to repay the state, leaving his heirs almost nothing.

As for Joe, his drinking takes its toll, and he also winds up in a nursing home. Since he is broke, he immediately qualifies for Medicaid, which pays all his bills. Upon his death, the state cannot be repaid since Joe leaves no estate. So, in essence, the government is content to pay all of John's hospital bills but wants Sam to first impoverish himself and then they take his house at his death, to pay for his nursing home bills. Meanwhile, Joe is rewarded for his profligate lifestyle by getting a free ride from the government; his family does not have to chip in one penny for his care.

Oh—there's one more guy we need to meet: Bob, who also managed to save up $100,000 and pay off his house, but who was a little more thoughtful than Sam and who hired an elder law attorney to give him advice. That lawyer was aware of all the provisions of the Medicaid rules and regulations, and advised Bob to make some loans, some approved purchases, and some gifts to family members, so that by the time Bob entered a nursing home, his assets were protected. Thus, Bob received the same care as Sam, but his assets were passed to his family and did not have to be spent on nursing home bills.

Is Sam, who managed to build up a small amount of savings, more ethical than Joe, who squandered his money and then had the government pay for his care? Is Sam more ethical than Bob, who simply followed the rules and regulations enacted by the state and federal government, and managed to protect his life savings and house? And how does that differ from the guy in the Lexus who pays top dollar to the Big Four accounting firm for clever tax planning, setting up offshore corporations so his business can legally avoid paying millions in income taxes? Legal, yes. Ethical? I leave that to you. But in any event, is it any more ethical than Medicaid planning?

As the great Judge Learned Hand famously said in the case of *Helvering v.*

Gregory (1934),

> *"Any one may so arrange his affairs that his taxes shall be as low as possible; he is not bound to choose that pattern which will best pay the Treasury; there is not even a patriotic duty to increase one's taxes. . . . Over and over again courts have said that there is nothing sinister in so arranging one's affairs as to keep taxes as low as possible. Everybody does so, rich or poor; and all do right, for nobody owes any public duty to pay more than the law demands: taxes are enforced exactions, not voluntary contributions. To demand more in the name of morals is mere cant."*

The United States Supreme Court reinforced this sentiment in affirming the above ruling:

> *"The legal right of a taxpayer to decrease the amount of what otherwise would be his taxes, or altogether avoid them, by means which the law permits, cannot be doubted."*

No one says you have to take advantage of every possible available legal planning technique if you don't want to. You can also decide not to claim, say, a charitable deduction that is legally available to you on your Form 1040 and pay more income tax than you are required to do. **But it is certainly not unethical simply to avail yourself of the laws as they were enacted by the government in order to minimize your expenditures on nursing home care, and pass those savings on to your children.** This book will show you exactly how you can do that.

Chapter 2

WHAT IS "MEDICAID"?

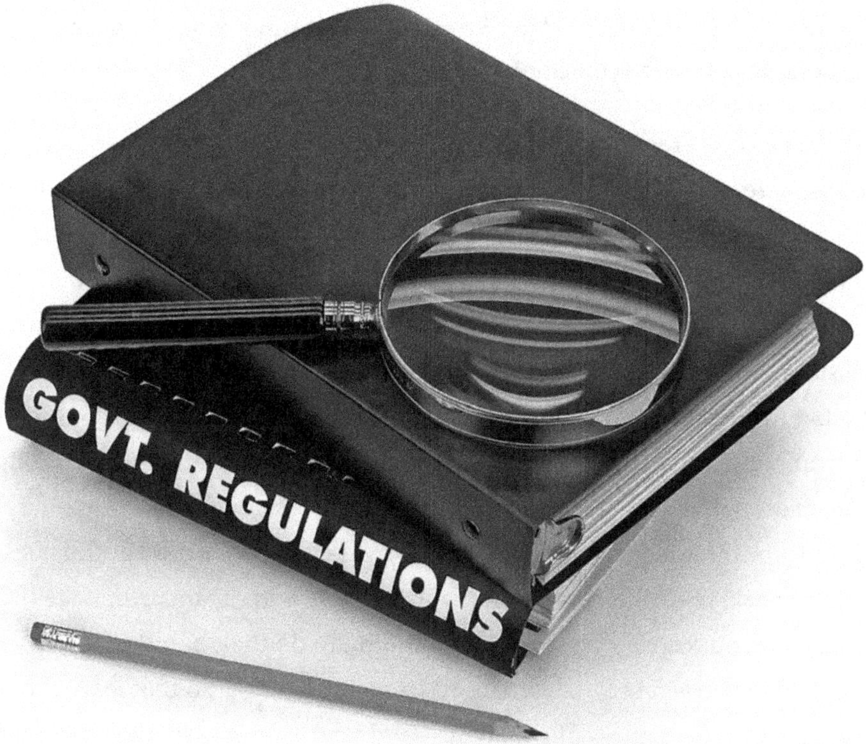

In brief,

Medicaid is a joint federal-state program for the medical care of certain needy populations within the United States. Although established by federal law, the Medicaid program is for the most part administered by the individual states. The cost is shared by the federal government and the states, with the federal government paying between 50% and 90% of the cost (it pays more to poorer states, less to the wealthier states).

What makes this area of the law so complicated is that under the federal statutes there are many options given to the states as to what they will pay for and who is entitled to coverage. As a result, you have 50 different versions of the Medicaid rules, with each state selecting a different combination of options, and each one interpreting the same laws differently. That leaves the residents of each state (including the lawyers, there!) scratching their heads trying to figure out what they can and cannot do, to qualify for Medicaid coverage. Unfortunately, you cannot simply ask the government for an advance ruling or interpretation, like you can with the IRS. That forces you to try something first and hope for the best. If you're challenged by the state Medicaid authorities, you can appeal their interpretation if you disagree with it, and even take them to court. Of course, very few people are willing to do that, because of the significant expense and hassle involved in such a lawsuit. So that leaves you relying on your best guess of what you—and your lawyer—think the state rules actually are.

Chapter 3

WHAT IS COVERED BY "MEDICAID"?

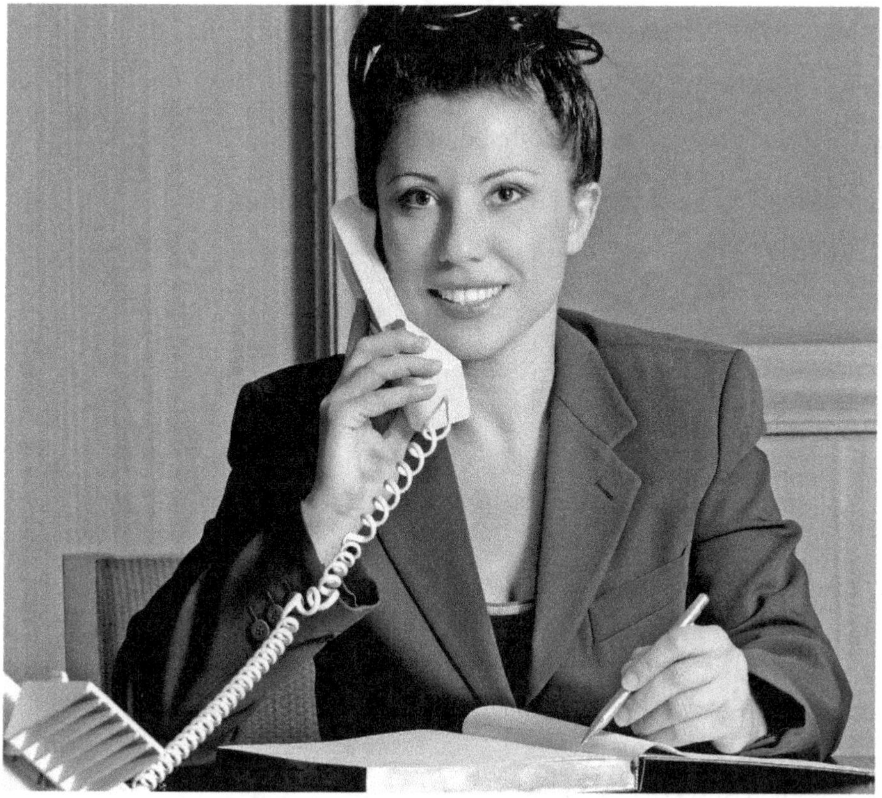

Medical Coverage

Once you have been approved for Medicaid, virtually all of your medical bills will be paid by the program. This includes your prescription drugs, hospital stays, nursing care, etc. Medicare may overlap this coverage, but one way or another your medical bills will be paid for you. Those who are receiving both Medicaid *and* Medicare coverage are known as "dual eligibles". Prescription drugs, formerly paid for by Medicaid, will now be paid for by Medicare Part D.

The following services *must* be offered by all states:

④ inpatient hospital services
④ outpatient hospital services
④ physician services
④ comprehensive dental services
④ nursing facility services for individuals age 21 or older
④ home health care for persons eligible for nursing facility services
④ lab and x-ray services
④ family nurse practitioner services

The following services are *optional*, but most states will offer them, also:

④ ambulatory services to individuals entitled to institutional care
④ home health services to individuals entitled to nursing facility services
④ prescribed drug coverage
④ optometrist services and eyeglasses
④ prosthetic devices
④ in-home assistance

What Is NOT Paid for by Medicaid (per Medicaid.gov)

④ Private room, unless medically needed
④ Specially prepared food, beyond that generally prepared by the facility
④ Telephone, television, radio

- Personal comfort items including tobacco products and confections
- Cosmetic and grooming items and services in excess of those included in the basic service
- Personal clothing
- Personal reading materials
- Gifts purchased on behalf of a resident
- Flowers and plants
- Social events and activities beyond the activity program
- Special care services not included in the facility's Medicaid payment

Care in Your Home

If you are living in your home, i.e., not in a nursing home, the Medicaid program refers to you as living "in the community," and Medicaid will still pay for certain services if you qualify. Many states have a program called "HCBS," which stands for "Home and Community Based Services." Until recently, a state wishing to provide Medicaid assistance to elderly people outside the nursing home had to apply to the federal government for a specific "waiver" of the usual Medicaid rules. Since 2007 states have been authorized to offer this program *without* first having to obtain a federal waiver. Hopefully, this will expand the access to HCBS nationally. In any event you must check to see if you qualify under your state's HCBS programs, which may be limited to certain geographic areas, certain types of disability, etc.

In general, HCBS will pay for the following in-home services:

- case management
- personal care services
- respite care services (i.e., care for the patient in a nursing home for a few days, to give the home caregiver a needed break)
- adult day health services
- homemaker/home health aide services

- habilitation (i.e., assists people in furthering their skills in the areas of mobility, social behaviors, self-care, basic safety, housekeeping, personal hygiene, health care, and financial management)

Beginning in 2007, states began to offer to those who are already in a nursing home the option of living in the community, allowing them the ability to interact with their family and community away from the institutional setting. They will be able to have the same level of care, and be covered by Medicaid. Be sure to check if your state has implemented this new program or plans to do so shortly.

The 2010 **Affordable Care Act** (so-called "**Obamacare**") does not affect the rules for in-nursing-home Medicaid. However, it does include a number of provisions that expand the reach of community-based care, such as HCBS discussed above. Specifically:

- The **Community First Choice** rule is a state option under Medicaid that provides states choosing to participate in this option a six percentage point increase in federal Medicaid matching funds for providing community-based attendant services and supports to people who would otherwise be confined to a nursing home or other institution. In other words, it encourages states to expand coverage to in-home care by offering them a financial incentive to do so.
- Under Section 2404 of the Affordable Care Act (ACA), the spousal impoverishment provisions that apply to couples where one spouse is in a nursing home (see discussion of the CSRA) will also apply to the well spouse in a couple where the other spouse is receiving HCBS. This provision is set to expire at the end of fiscal year 2027.
- The **Independence at Home Demonstration**—which is voluntary for Medicare patients—provides chronically ill Medicare patients with a complete range of in-home primary care services. Under the Demonstration, the Centers for Medicare & Medicaid Services (CMS) will partner with primary care practices led by physicians or nurse practitioners to evaluate the extent to which delivering primary care

services in a home setting is effective in improving care for Medicare patients with multiple chronic conditions and in reducing costs.

Assisted Living

In most states, it is possible to have Medicaid pay for certain services even if you are living in an assisted living facility. These are under the HCBS program described above. Note that the facility must be "Medicaid certified," so you will want to make sure about that when you are searching for a facility to move into. Note, however, that the facility's cost of basic room and board will *not* be paid for by Medicaid, as it would be if you resided in a nursing home.

Nursing Homes

Medicaid will pay the full nursing home bill, including room, board, and all nursing care costs.

However, it is very important to note that although 62% of all nursing home beds in the United States are filled with patients on the Medicaid program, not every nursing home accepts Medicaid payments. Thus, it is extremely important that you find out before you sign up for a nursing home whether it accepts Medicaid patients. While it is against the law for a nursing home to evict you because you run out of money and must go from private pay to Medicaid, that does not apply if the nursing home does not accept Medicaid from anyone! Be sure to ask! It is very upsetting to the nursing home resident to have to relocate from one nursing home to another, after finally accepting the fact that they are in a nursing home for good, have gotten used to the routines, made friends, become acquainted with the nurses, etc.

You may be worried that your family member will be less well-treated in a nursing home if the staff knows they are on Medicaid vs. paying privately. It may assuage you to know that there is a specific federal regulation that requires nursing homes to have the identical policies and practices regarding the provision of services for all residents "regardless of the source of payment."

Indeed, the staff generally has no idea which beds hold Medicaid patients vs. private pay patients.

Medicare Coverage of Nursing Home Expenses

Many people are under the mistaken impression that Medicare will cover their long-term nursing home stays. Here are the rules:

In order for Medicare to cover a person's nursing home stay, the patient must:

1. Have been hospitalized for medically necessary **inpatient hospital care** for **at least 3 consecutive days**, not counting the date of discharge,
2. Be **admitted** to the nursing home **within 30 days** after the date of discharge from the hospital,
3. Require **skilled** nursing or rehab care on a daily basis for a condition for which the patient was hospitalized, and
4. Receive **a physician's order** that such care is needed.

Skilled Care. Skilled care is care that can only be administered by professional (physician or nurse) or technical personnel and which will prevent further deterioration in the patient's health. Examples are intravenous feeding, injections, insertion of catheters, application of sterile dressings, treatment of skin ulcers, and therapeutic exercises of various kinds. Less medically intensive and critical personal care services, even if done by a nurse, are not considered skilled care. Note that it is not necessary that the care result in the patient's condition improving; skilled care may also be needed to keep the patient from regressing and to preserve their current status. For a long time there was some dispute about this, but it was finally settled by law in 2013 to indicate that such improvement is not a condition of receiving Medicare coverage.

Custodial Care. If the care of the patient does not require "skilled care" as defined above, such care is called "custodial care." This is the type of long-term care typically rendered in a nursing home. As stated above, the mere fact that a patient's condition does not "improve" does not change otherwise "skilled care" into "custodial care."

100-Day Limit. Once in the nursing home, the patient will only be covered by Medicare for a *maximum* of 100 days during any benefit period (also referred to as a "spell of illness"). Such benefit period means a period of consecutive days beginning with the first day (not included in a previous benefit period) on which a patient is admitted to a hospital (or other covered facility)— and which occurs in a month for which he or she is entitled to Medicare Part A benefits— and ending with the close of the first period of 60 consecutive days thereafter on each of which the patient is neither an inpatient of a hospital nor an inpatient of a nursing facility. In other words, to determine the 60-consecutive-day period, begin counting with the day the patient was discharged. If the patient is not re-admitted within the next 60 days, then a new benefit period can begin. A person may be discharged from and readmitted to a hospital or skilled nursing facility several times during a single benefit period and still be in the same benefit period if 60 consecutive days have not elapsed between discharge and readmission. Furthermore, the stays need not be for related physical or mental conditions.

Co-Pay Rule. Finally, even if the patient manages to qualify for Medicare coverage of their nursing home stay, Medicare only fully pays the bill for days 1-20. For days 21-100, Medicare requires the patient to pay the "SNF care coinsurance" amount, which in 2025 is $209.50 per day (set annually by the federal government).

Example:

Charles, over age 65, is admitted to the hospital on March 1. He is entitled to Medicare coverage under Part A (which covers hospitalization costs). On March 5 he is moved to a skilled nursing facility, but his condition improves and he is sent home on April 1. (From March 5 through March 24, Medicare paid the entire nursing home bill; from March 25 to April 1, Charles had a copayment of $209.50 per day.) After a few weeks, his condition worsens and he is re-admitted to the hospital on May 1 and the nursing facility on May 3. He remains in the nursing facility until July 30, requiring skilled care. His nursing facility Medicare coverage picks up where his last coverage left off (i.e., with day 29), so he is required to pay the co-pay from May 3 through July 14. At that point, his "100 days of coverage per benefit period" expires, and he will have to pay the nursing facility the full amount of its bill from July 15 to July 30 (unless, of course, he has private insurance that will cover him). Because Charles was absent from a hospital or nursing facility for fewer than 60 days (April 1-May 1), he is still within his initial benefit period.

NOTE: Although Charles was discharged from the nursing home and was later re-admitted, there is no requirement the second time that he first be admitted to a hospital for three consecutive days in order to be covered by Medicare, like there was the first time. His coverage days pick up where they left off, since he is still within the same benefit period. If instead he had been re-admitted after May 31 (i.e., more than 60 days after he left the facility), then a new 100-day period of coverage would apply, and again for the first 20 days there would be no co-payment due, then a co-payment due for days 21-100, etc.

Chapter 4

APPLYING FOR BENEFITS

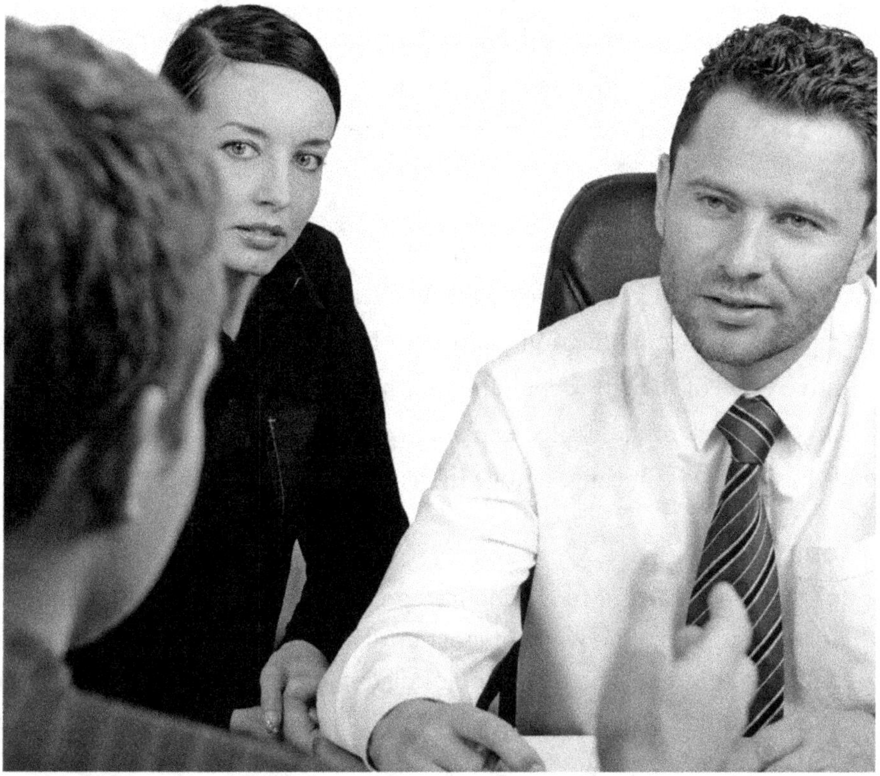

When to Apply

Applying Too Late

Applying too late can mean that the opportunity to have the government pay for your family member's care will be lost, costing your family thousands of dollars. Although in most states it is permissible to apply for benefits for the period starting up to three months prior to the date of application, you cannot go back any further than that (see *Retroactive Coverage*). Thus, it makes sense to apply as soon as you are sure your family member can qualify.

Applying Too Early

Applying too early can be a very expensive mistake if gifts have been made that affect eligibility! Most gifts made by the Medicaid applicant and/or spouse can cause a period of disqualification if either or both of them apply for Medicaid within five years of the gift (depending on the date made; see *Transferring Assets* in Chapter 8 for a detailed explanation). Applying before this "lookback period" has expired can cause a huge increase in the penalty period.

Example:

John made a transfer to his children on March 1, 2020, of his house, worth $250,000. If he waits at least until March 1, 2025 to apply for Medicaid, there will be no period of disqualification, because his gift was made outside of the five-year lookback period. However, if he applies for Medicaid on February 1, 2025, he could be disqualified from receiving Medicaid coverage for 50 months or more (depending on what state he lives in)!

Sometimes it makes sense to apply during the lookback period because you want to get the penalty period running. This technique is explained in more detail in Chapter 14 under the *Half-a-Loaf* discussion).

So the rule is, never apply until you're sure your family member qualifies, or if you are certain you want the penalty period to start immediately. In any event, if any gifts have been made within the last

five years, the opinion of an experienced elder law attorney should be sought prior to actually applying for Medicaid, to make sure the time is right to do so.

Who Can Apply?

The individual seeking to receive Medicaid benefits may themselves be the applicant. However, usually it will be a family member who applies on behalf of the potential Medicaid recipient. The person named under a power of attorney may also apply, as may a court-appointed guardian. Indeed, the applicant may appoint any individual to assist with the application, renewal, and ongoing communication with the Medicaid agency. Since January 1, 2014, federal regulations allow an applicant to name an *organization* to apply on behalf of the applicant, as well. Thus, the nursing home itself is permitted fill out the application form and assist with the application, if designated by the Medicaid applicant.

Where to Apply

Every state has a system in place to permit you to apply for Medicaid benefits. The best way to find out where you need to go is to contact the state Medicaid Agency in your state.

List of State Agencies

For a list of state agencies that supervise the application process, see the following: https://aq-iq.com/state-medicaid-agencies-provider-directory/.

Application Process

The application form will require you to list your current income and assets. You will also need to bring in your bank account records going back anywhere from six months to as much as five years. You may have to provide copies of deeds, trusts, and insurance policies. Some states are now requiring Medicaid applicants to produce a copy of every check that they have written in the last five years. Checks written as a Christmas gift, Easter gift, birthday gift, or church donation, could be cause for the applicant to be disqualified. However, if the gifts were made *exclusively* for a purpose *other than to qualify for Medicaid*, the gifts must be ignored. Thus, it is a good idea to start gathering the necessary information in advance of your application. Otherwise, your inability to provide the necessary documents or information could result in the imposition of a penalty period for such gifts; at the least, it could cause a delay in the processing of your application, which in turn could cause you to lose valuable benefits.

Retroactive Coverage

It may be possible to apply for Medicaid coverage for a period beginning up to three months prior to the date of application. If the applicant *would have* qualified for Medicaid as of such date had he or she applied at such time, then the applicant will be covered starting on such date. (A state may even cover the applicant as of the first day of that month.) For example, if you thought you would not qualify for Medicaid for several months and then found out you actually *could have* qualified, you can apply for Medicaid immediately, and ask for coverage going back up to three months. Unfortunately, the period of time before the three-month date will not be covered by Medicaid, even if you could have qualified had you applied back then. Thus it is very important to apply as soon as you are qualified; once that three-month retroactive window closes, your family may wind up having to pay privately for your care when you *could* have gotten Medicaid to pay all of your nursing home expenses.

> NOTE: As of January 1, 2025, at least 11 states (Arizona, Delaware, Florida, Indiana, Kentucky, New Hampshire, Maine, Massachusetts, New Mexico, Oklahoma, and Utah) have eliminated or restricted the right of a person in a nursing home to obtain retroactive coverage or have applied for a federal waiver to do so. As just mentioned, the general rule under

federal law is to permit three months retroactive coverage. However, these states have either obtained or applied for a waiver to deviate from this federal requirement.

IMPORTANT: Thus, to be on the safe side, be sure to apply for Medicaid as soon as possible—which may even be *before* admission to a nursing home in some cases—assuming the applicant would otherwise qualify!

Documentation of Citizenship

Since July 1, 2006, anyone applying for or receiving Medicaid needs to prove that they are either a U.S. citizen or national or a qualified alien. Such proof must be made at the time of applying for Medicaid for the first time, or upon the first redetermination of eligibility (which is done once a year following initial approval) for those already receiving Medicaid coverage. It is only done once per person.

Such proof may only be made by one or more of the following:

- U.S. passport
- Certificate of Naturalization (Form N-550 or N-570)
- Certificate of U. S. Citizenship (Form N-560 or N-561)
- A valid state-issued driver's license or ID document BUT ONLY if the state requires proof of U.S. citizenship prior to issuance or obtains and verifies the individual's Social Security Number
- If none of the above is available, then the applicant can provide any of the following to establish citizenship:
- U.S. birth certificate
- Other evidence of U.S. citizenship if born abroad, adopted, etc.
- If none of the above is available, there are still other methods allowed, in rare circumstances, such as hospital records, census records, medical records, and written affidavit if all else fails.
- If one of the first four methods listed above cannot be used, then the applicant must also submit one of the following to establish identity:

- ④ A valid state-issued driver's license with photo or other identifying information
- ④ School. ID card with photo
- ④ U.S. military card or draft record
- ④ Government ID. card with photo or other ID information
- ④ All copies must either be originals or copies certified by the issuing agency; notarized copies are not acceptable.
- ④ Such other documentation as the Secretary of Health and Human Services may allow, by regulation. For complete details, you can search online for "Medicaid citizenship guidelines" to find the final rules issued by the Centers for Medicare & Medicaid Services (CMS).

Because it may take some time to obtain the above documentation, particularly if one of the first four methods of proof is unavailable, the family should assist the prospective Medicaid applicant in getting this documentation together as soon as possible.

Nursing Home Bills Before You Are on Medicaid

Whether or not you are already Medicaid eligible will affect initial nursing home charges. If you are not yet Medicaid eligible, because you have to spend down first or you have a penalty period to wait out, a nursing home is legally allowed to require you to pay a deposit or sign a promissory note in order to be admitted. In addition, they may want to be satisfied that you have sufficient funds to pay privately for at least a few months (such funds are sometimes referred to as "key money"). Because nursing homes make more money from residents who privately pay than those on Medicaid, and they typically have a limited number of beds set aside for Medicaid patients, you may find yourself on a long waiting list to get into your nursing home of choice unless you can at least enter as a private-pay resident. Accordingly, when doing your Medicaid planning, be careful not to give *everything* away, leaving yourself completely broke and therefore potentially unable to get into your nursing home of choice. It is for this reason that many attorneys recommend that as part of your

Medicaid asset protection plan you retain at least enough funds to pay privately for your first three to six months in a nursing home; when those funds run out—if you've planned properly—you can apply for Medicaid. (Don't worry—a nursing home cannot legally evict you for switching from private pay to Medicaid pay.)

What happens if you applied for Medicaid but you are not yet qualified because you are waiting for the eligibility determination by the state? According to the CMS (Centers for Medicare & Medicaid Services), **a nursing facility is permitted to charge an applicant or resident whose Medicaid eligibility is pending,** typically in the form of a deposit prior to admission and/or payment for services after admission. The facility can charge you its regular private-pay rate, even though it will only be reimbursed by the state at the "Medicaid reimbursement rate." (The "Medicaid reimbursement rate" is the rate that the state pays the nursing home for each Medicaid resident, which is usually around 70% of the nursing home's private-pay rate.)

Interestingly, the CMS State Operation Manual indicates that if the nursing home, following the above rule, attempts to charge the resident during the Medicaid-pending period, and the resident does not pay, the nursing home may not evict the resident for non-payment. So the nursing home is allowed to bill during this period but may not enforce it! Since it can be difficult and time-consuming (and perhaps impossible without a lawsuit) to get the nursing home to refund money you already paid them, you should always hold off on paying them during the initial application period to the extent you can. (See *Nursing Home Eviction Rules*, Chapter 14).

In any event, once you are determined to be Medicaid-eligible, the payments you made to the nursing home during the Medicaid-pending period by law must be refunded to you (but may not be without filing a law suit), less the amount the state determines is your "share-of-costs" of your monthly nursing home bills (see *Patient's Share-of-Costs*, Chapter 15). Since you can be eligible up to three months prior to the date you file your Medicaid application

(*Retroactive Coverage*), all of your payments during those three months (less your share-of-costs amount) must be refunded to you.

Example:

Martha entered the Manor Rest Nursing Home on January 1, with $29,000 in the bank and no other assets. Her income is $1,000 per month from Social Security. She is not married and would have qualified for Medicaid except that she had $27,000 too much cash. In January, February, and March, she paid the nursing home its $10,000/month private-pay rate: $1,000 from her income and the balance ($9,000) out of her bank account.

By April 1 she only had $2,000 left in the bank. She could have qualified for Medicaid immediately at this point, but her family didn't get around to applying on her behalf until July 1. Since Martha could have qualified for Medicaid had she applied on April 1, her family requested that her coverage start on that date, under the "retroactive coverage" rule discussed above. On Sept. 1 Martha was approved for Medicaid, effective April 1. But until September 1 Martha still had to pay the nursing home its private pay rate, since she was not yet approved for Medicaid. So for April through August her family continued to pay the nursing home its $10,000/month charge, with Martha contributing her $1,000/month income and the family paying the balance of $9,000 per month out of their own pockets. Starting Sept. 1, of course, Medicaid will begin paying Martha's entire nursing home bill (at the facility's particular Medicaid reimbursement rate of $5,000/month, reduced by the monthly contribution of her $1,000 Social Security income).

Result: Starting Sept. 1, Manor Rest will owe Martha's family a total of $45,000: $9,000 a month for April, May, June, July, and August. (Manor Rest doesn't have to refund the full $10,000/month paid to them during this period, because Martha's $1,000/month income would go to them even under Medicaid, so those payments are not refunded.) The state will reimburse the nursing home $4,000/month for April through August (i.e., the $5,000 Medicaid reimbursement rate less Martha's "share of cost" contribution). From Sept. 1 on, the nursing home will receive

Medicaid reimbursement of $4,000/month from the state so long as Martha continues to reside there.

Fortunately, some nursing homes will not charge a patient who has applied for Medicaid during the Medicaid-pending period. If the application is initially denied, though, then all the back payments must be made up, and regular monthly payments must start. If you appeal the denial, some nursing homes will want to be paid during the appeal; others will wait until after the appeal is resolved.

Be aware that some states have a rule that a Medicaid applicant is not eligible for coverage in any month that the nursing home has been paid in full. Perhaps the state's rationale is that there was no need for Medicaid, since the bill was fully paid, so they will not extend eligibility for any such month. Accordingly, in such states, it is important that the nursing home be paid somewhat less than the amount it bills you, to avoid this problem. The billing office in the nursing home will undoubtedly have run into this before so it should not be an issue with them. They will either be reimbursed by the state once you're approved (assuming they received at least the Medicaid reimbursement rate), or there will be a small amount due them if you're denied, which your family will have to pay.

If the nursing home does not require payment during the Medicaid-pending period, and then later you are approved, the nursing home (or your elder law attorney) will be able to apply to Medicaid for reimbursement. But you will still be required to pay the monthly patient "share-of-costs" amount (see *Patient's Share-of-Costs*, Chapter 15) If you are not ultimately approved for Medicaid, obviously you will owe all the back charges to the nursing home, at their private-pay rate.

Filial Responsibility Laws

Under the laws of 25 states, a child has the legal obligation to support their parents if the parents are unable to do so themselves, to the extent of the child's ability to do so. In most states these “filial responsibility” laws have not been enforced for many years: once Medicare, Social Security, and Medicaid were enacted to offer a safety net to seniors, these laws were less important.

However, there have been a few very recent cases that relied on such statutes to require a child to pay the nursing home bill of their parent; one case, in Pennsylvania, required the son to pay his mother’s $93,000 nursing home bill! On the other hand, at least one very recent court case has held that such statutes do not apply in this situation, pointing to the federal statutes that prohibit a nursing home from requiring a third party to guarantee payment to the facility as a condition of admission and holding that such statutes trump the state filial support law. Regardless of the law in your state, once the parent is eligible for Medicaid, the child is “off the hook” as far as the nursing home bill is concerned, so it is further incentive for a child to do proper Medicaid planning for a parent!

Chapter 5

MEDICAL QUALIFICATION RULES

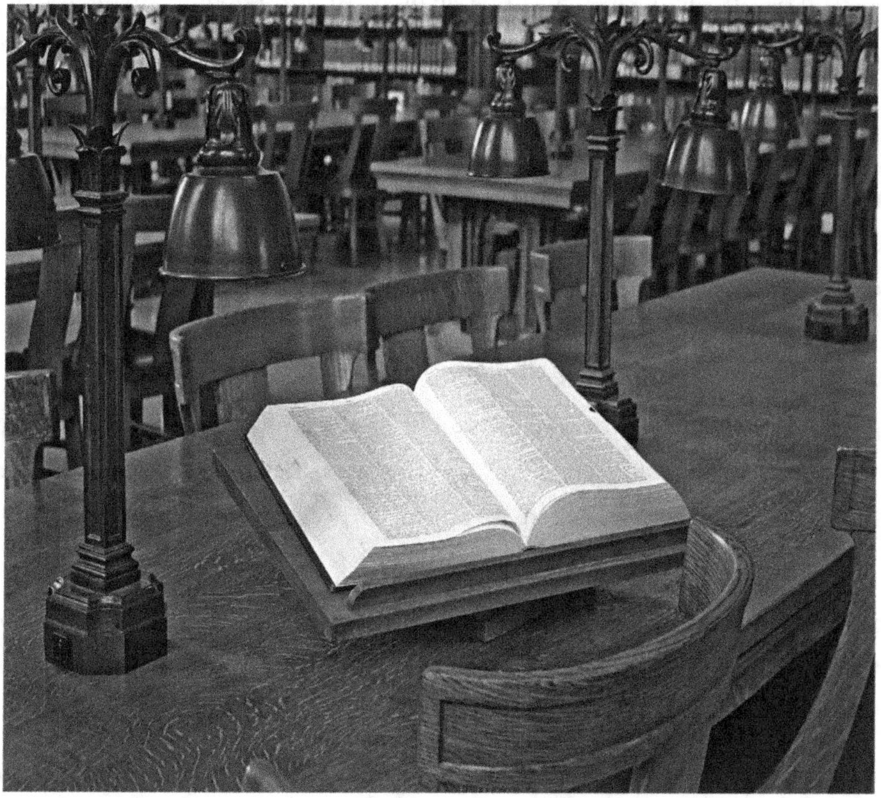

In addition to the strict financial rules that are the focus of this book, there are also medical qualifications to meet before a person will be eligible for Medicaid coverage for a nursing home stay. The applicant must prove he or she is at least age 65, blind, or disabled. According to the federal regulations, to be disabled means that you are unable "to do any substantial gainful activity by reason of any medically determinable physical or mental impairment that can be expected to result in death or which has lasted or can be expected to last for a continuous period of not less than 12 months."

Typically, the state will send a nurse or trained intake worker to the Medicaid applicant's home, to interview the applicant. The nurse or worker will have a checklist of Activities of Daily Living (ADLs) and in order to be deemed "sick" enough to qualify for Medicaid, the applicant must "fail" a certain number of these tests. Thus, this is not a time for the applicant to downplay his or her disabilities; such comments can cause the nurse or worker to think the applicant is actually in better shape than he or she really is, with the result that Medicaid coverage will be denied. If that happens, the applicant's only recourse at that point is to begin an expensive appeals process.

Meeting the medical qualifications is not typically an issue when you are looking at a frail elderly or Alzheimer's patient. The real issues are more often that of having too much income or too many assets, so let's move on and take a detailed look at that.

Chapter 6

INCOME QUALIFICATION RULES

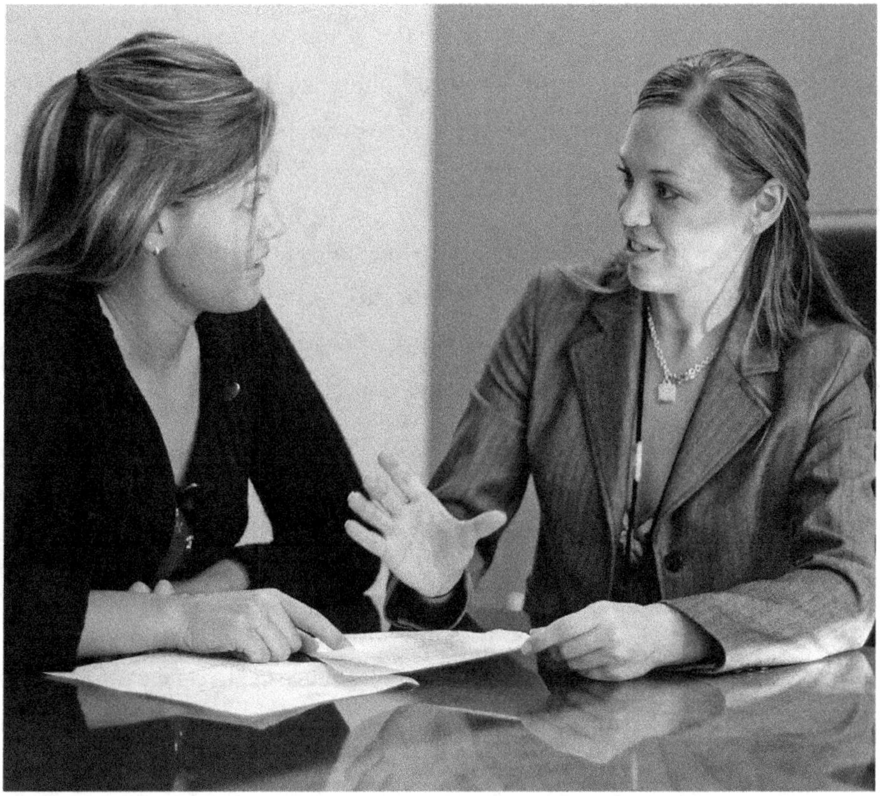

Unmarried

An unmarried individual may not have more than $2,901 of income per month. (This 2025 figure, published by the federal government, changes annually to reflect cost-of-living changes.) "Income" for these purposes includes both "earned" income (wages) and "unearned" income (interest and dividends).

What if your income exceeds this amount? There are actually two different ways this is handled, depending on the state in which you live.

"Income-cap" States

At the time of this writing, only the following states are "income-cap" states: Alabama, Alaska, Arizona, Arkansas, Colorado, Delaware, Florida, Georgia, Idaho, Indiana, Iowa, Kentucky, Mississippi, Nevada, New Jersey, New Mexico, Oklahoma, Oregon, South Carolina, South Dakota, Tennessee, Texas, and Wyoming.

In an "income-cap" state, if your income is even one dollar above the limit, you are initially disqualified from Medicaid. That's not a problem if the state is also a "medically needy" state, which means that you can still qualify by deducting your medical expenses (including nursing home costs) to get your income below the limit. But in the other states, a problem arises if you earn too much money to qualify for Medicaid to help you pay the nursing home bill, but not enough to pay for it privately!

It was this exact dilemma that led to the lawsuit that finally created the solution: all these other states now allow you to set up a simple trust and have your income paid to the trust. The trust then takes the income and pays it to the nursing home each month. This type of trust is known as a "Qualified Income Trust" or "Miller Trust" (after the case, *Miller v. Ibarra*, that established this trust procedure). A family member can act as the trustee of this trust, keeping the costs down. Assuming you follow some basic rules about this process, your excess income will not prevent you from qualifying for Medicaid, unless your income exceeds the actual cost of the nursing home. Of course, in this case since the entire nursing home bill is being paid out of your income, there would really be no need for Medicaid assistance. It is important to note that excess income must be transferred monthly in order for an Medicaid recipient to remain eligible and ONLY income can be placed in a Qualified Income Trust. This type of trust cannot be used to shelter excess assets.

For the most recent Medicaid Eligibility Income chart by state visit https://www.medicaidplanningassistance.org/medicaid-eligibility-income-chart/

In each of the following examples, assume that the individual applying for Medicaid is single, is already in a nursing home, and has minimal assets.

Example 1:

Sam has only his Social Security income of $900/month to live on. He will qualify for Medicaid. Each month his Social Security check goes to the nursing home, and Medicaid picks up the balance of his bill.

Example 2:

Martin has Social Security income of $1,800 and a small monthly pension of $1,400. He will also qualify for Medicaid, but since his total income of $3,200 exceeds $2,901 (the income upper limit to avoid needing a trust), a Qualified Income Trust will have to be set up to receive either his Social Security income or his pension; this will reduce his countable income below the limit. That income is then paid over to the nursing home, and once again Medicaid will pay the balance of the bill.

Example 3:

Mary has Social Security, a pension, and some oil lease income that together total $8,000 per month. In the state where Mary lives, that's actually more than the cost of her monthly nursing home bill, so she will not qualify for Medicaid because her income is just too high. Is there a way for her to reduce her income? She is unable to assign her Social Security or pension to another family member, since those are non-assignable under the law. However, she can probably assign her oil lease interest, which would carry the income with it to the new owner. Of course, such assignment is a gift and will cause a penalty period (see discussion of gifts, Chapter 8). However, it is an option that should be considered and discussed with the elder law attorney who will assist Mary to qualify for Medicaid.

Spenddown ("Medically Needy") States

The balance of the states permit the nursing home resident to spend down his or her monthly income (on medical expenses and, most of these states provide, on nursing home costs), with Medicaid paying the shortfall. In other words, so long as the income of the applicant is below the actual cost of the nursing home, the applicant can qualify for Medicaid (assuming the applicant also meets the asset test).

Married

The treatment of income of a married couple is vastly more complicated than that of a single individual. That is because of the various attribution rules that permit the income of the nursing home spouse to be shifted to the spouse still residing in the community (i.e., the "Community Spouse"). As a result of this opportunity, there is much planning that can be done to maximize the income of the Community Spouse and minimize the income of the nursing home spouse.

The first rule to remember about the treatment of income when one spouse of a married couple applies for Medicaid is "the name on the check determines whose income it is." So a payment of annuity or pension income to one spouse is deemed that spouse's income only, and a check payable to both is deemed paid 50% to each spouse.

Note that the "name on the check" rule applies only to checks from a company or asset not owned by the spouses, e.g., a check from a pension or Social Security, or from employment. Income from an asset owned solely by one spouse is deemed that spouse's income. Income from assets owned by both spouses (i.e., in some form of joint ownership) will be attributed to the spouses in equal shares, unless the controlling document (if any) specifically allocates the income otherwise. This applies to jointly owned interests in real estate, bank accounts, corporate stock, LLC, partnership, promissory note, annuity, etc. Note that this is a rebuttable presumption: for example, if indeed all of the money in a joint account can be traced to the contribution of one spouse, then it should be possible to prove that the account income should be deemed to be only that of the contributing spouse. If the ownership interest in the income itself can be proved to be other than the general rules set forth above, then that supersedes the general rules. Payments from a trust also follow the "name on the check" rule unless the trust document allocates the income in some other manner.

Example:

Alice receives $350 a month from a rental property she owns jointly with her husband, Bill. Each month the tenant makes the check out to Alice, only. Nonetheless, because the property is owned jointly by Alice and Bill, the income generated by that property is divided equally between them. So even though the check is only payable to Alice, Medicaid will still deem 50% of the monthly rent—$175—to be Bill's income.

The important point to remember is that if you are living in the community and your spouse is in the nursing home, you will not have to contribute any portion of your income toward your spouse's nursing home bill, under the Medicaid rules.

Example:

Joe, who is still living at home, has pension and Social Security income totaling $2,500/month. His wife, Edie, now resides in a nursing home. Her income is only from Social Security and equals only $450/month. Nonetheless, Joe does *not* have to contribute one penny to Edie's nursing home care, once she is approved for Medicaid, and he can keep his entire $2,500 each month.

"Income-cap" States

For married couples in an "income-cap" state (see discussion on "Income-cap" States in Chapter 6), you must first look at the gross income of the applicant spouse. If it's over the state maximum, a Qualified Income Trust must be established for the benefit of the applicant spouse. However, the trust can then pay the personal needs allowance, the spousal protected amount (MMMNA), the family allowance, and non-covered medical expenses. Although the income in the trust is not counted for Medicaid purposes, if the total net income of the applicant spouse (after all these deductions) exceeds the actual cost of the nursing home then the applicant will not qualify for Medicaid. Of course, in this case since the entire nursing home bill is being paid out of the nursing home spouse's income, there would really be no need for Medicaid assistance.

MIA/MMMNA Rules

Although the Community Spouse never has to contribute any of his or her income to the other spouse's care, it is possible for the nursing home spouse's income to be paid to the Community Spouse. So it's a one-way street: income only flows—if at all—from the nursing home spouse to the Community Spouse, and never vice versa.

That's because the Community Spouse is entitled to a minimum monthly income of between $2,555 and $3,853 (depending on the state; for the income limits for your state, go to https://www.medicaidplanningassistance.org/state-specific-medicaid-eligibility/ and click on your state name.) These figures are set by the federal government and change annually. The applicable figure for the particular state is known as the "Minimum Monthly Maintenance Needs Allowance" or "MMMNA." If the Community Spouse's income is less than the MMMNA, then a certain amount of the nursing home spouse's income may be allocated to the Community Spouse, sufficient (to the extent possible) to increase the Community Spouse's income up to the MMMNA. Such allotment of income from the nursing home spouse to the Community Spouse is called the Monthly Income Allowance, or "MIA."

Example 1:

Assume the Community Spouse has no income other than $500 a month from Social Security, and the nursing home spouse has Social Security of $1,000 a month. Based on these numbers, the amount of the nursing home spouse's income that can be shifted over to the Community Spouse—the MIA—will be $1,055 which is more than the nursing home spouse's income amount. The Community Spouse will be entitled to keep all the couple's combined income, because the total of their combined income would be only $1,500 per month. Since that's less than the minimum entitlement income of $2,555, the Community Spouse can keep all of the income, and Medicaid will pay the entire nursing home bill.

MMMNA	**$2,555**
Community Spouse's income Shortfall	**(500)**
	2,055
Nursing home spouse's income	**1,000**
Amount able to be shifted (MIA)	**1,000**

NOTE: You can never shift more than the lesser of the shortfall figure or the total amount of the nursing home spouse's income. If the nursing home spouse's income is less than the shortfall amount, it may be possible to increase the amount of excluded assets the Community Spouse can retain.

See Increasing the CSRA, Chapter 7.

Example 2:

Assume the Community Spouse has income of $1000 a month, and the nursing home spouse has income of $2,000 a month. Based on these numbers, the Community Spouse will be allowed to keep $1,555 from the nursing home spouse's income, i.e., an MIA of $1,555 (which brings the Community Spouse up to $2,555). The nursing home spouse will then contribute the balance of his or her income ($2,000 – $1,555 = $455) every month toward the nursing home bill. Medicaid will pick up the balance of the bill.

MMMNA	**$2,555**
Community Spouse's income shortfall	**(1000)**
	1,555
Nursing home spouse's income	**2,000**
Amount able to be shifted (MIA)	**1,555**
Amount to be paid to nursing home from nursing home spouse's income= $445	

NOTE: You can never shift more than the shortfall figure.

Example 3:

Assume the Community Spouse has income of $2,600 a month, and the nursing home spouse has income of $500 a month. In this case, because the Community Spouse's income exceeds the MMMNA of $2,555, no portion of the nursing home spouse's income is allowed to be shifted to the Community Spouse. As a result, the nursing home spouse must pay all of his or her monthly income toward the nursing home bill, and Medicaid will pick up the balance of the bill, once the nursing home spouse has qualified for Medicaid coverage.

MMMNA	**$2,555**
Community Spouse's income Shortfall	**(2,600)**

	-0-
Nursing home spouse's income	**500**
Amount able to be shifted (MIA)	**-0-**

Increasing the MMMNA

Sometimes it is possible to increase the income of the Community Spouse above the minimum amount (MMMNA), although in no case can a state permit an increase above $3,853.50 without either a court order of support or proof that the Community Spouse would face "significant financial duress" due to "exceptional circumstances."

There are three ways to do this: increase the MMMNA by the amount of the Excess Shelter Allowance, apply for a Fair Hearing, or obtain a court order of support for the Community Spouse.

Excess Shelter Allowance (ESA)

In a state with an MMMNA less than the absolute maximum permitted under federal law ($3,853.50), it may be possible to increase the MMMNA based on high "shelter" costs. If the "shelter" costs of the Community Spouse exceed 30% of the MMMNA, then this excess may be added on top of the MMMNA, but only up to the maximum monthly allowance figure published by the federal government (currently $3,853.50). Since the current MMMNA is $2,555, 30% of that is $766.50. So if the shelter costs of the Community Spouse exceed $766.50, that excess amount may be added to the MMMNA when trying to figure out how much of the nursing home spouse's income can be shifted over to the Community Spouse.

For these purposes, "shelter" expenses only include rent or mortgage payment, condo fees (if any), real estate taxes and homeowner's insurance, and either the standard utility allowance (currently between $266 and $848, depending on the state) or, if your state does not use such an allowance, the actual cost of utilities (heat, electricity, gas, and—in most states—telephone service). Some states even permit you to use the higher of the standard utility allowance or actual cost of utilities when calculating whether or not you qualify for the Excess Shelter Allowance. Once again, you need to check your own state's regulations on this point.

In those few states where the standard utility allowance by itself exceeds the standard shelter allowance, the MMMNA will always be increased, at least by the amount of that excess.

Example:

Mary lives at home in the community, and her husband, Joe, is in the nursing home. Mary's income is $1,114 a month, all from Social Security. Joe's monthly income is $2,500, from his Social Security and pension. Because Mary's income is less than $2,555, we know she is entitled to shift a portion of Joe's income to her. Ignoring shelter costs, she is entitled to $2,555 – $1,114, or $1441.

MMMNA	**$2,555**
Community Spouse's income Shortfall	**(1,114)**
	1441
Nursing home spouse's income	**2,500**
Amount able to be shifted (MIA)	**$1441**

NOTE: You can never shift more than the shortfall figure.

Because Joe has excess income even after he shifts some of it to Mary, we should try to see if there's a way to increase the amount Mary is entitled to. After all, Joe's income will all have to go to the nursing home, where it won't do him any good: it will simply reduce the amount that Medicaid would otherwise pay the nursing home. So the next step is to see if Mary would be entitled to more of Joe's income if her shelter costs are high enough. Here are the figures:

Condo fees	**$250**
Real estate taxes	**150**
Homeowner's insurance	**100**
Standard Utility Allowance	**375**
TOTAL:	**875**
Shelter allowance	**(400)**
	$475
Excess Shelter Allowance	

Because her shelter costs ($875) exceed the standard shelter allowance ($400), Mary is allowed to add the excess ($875–$400 = $475) to the MMMNA ($2,555) for an increased MMMNA of $3,030 ($2,555 + $475). Since her own income is $1,114, this means she is entitled to shift $1,916 ($3,030 - $1,114) from Joe's income to herself, each month. Joe's contribution to the nursing home each month will now be reduced by the same amount that is shifted over to Mary. This process allows Mary to keep an additional $5,700 of Joe's income each year!

Summary:

MMMNA	**$2,555**
Excess Shelter Allowance (ESA)	**475**
Increased MMMNA	**3,030**
Community Spouse's income	**1114**
Shortfall	**(1,441)**

Nursing home spouse's income	2,500
Amount able to be shifted (MIA)	1,916
Amount paid to nursing home from nursing home spouse's income= $584	

Borrowing to Increase the ESA and MMMNA

As discussed above, most states have both a minimum Monthly Maintenance Needs Allowance (MMMNA) and a maximum MMMNA. In such states it is possible to increase the amount of income allocated to the Community Spouse by increasing shelter costs so they exceed the Excess Shelter Allowance This would apply when the nursing home spouse has income from Social Security or a pension, the Community Spouse has income of less than the maximum MMMNA, and there is a home titled solely in the name of the Community Spouse.

First, the Community Spouse takes out a loan against the home's equity. Assuming the nursing home spouse has already been approved for Medicaid, this extra cash will not disqualify the nursing home spouse as long as it is deposited into an account owned solely by the Community Spouse. The new mortgage payments are excess shelter costs, and any payment over the shelter standard will therefore increase the amount of income the Community Spouse is entitled to shift from the nursing home spouse, up to the maximum MMMNA ($3,853.50/month). To get the mortgage payment as high as possible, the Community Spouse should consider a very short payback period. The length of the payback period will depend on the amount of additional income able to be shifted from the nursing home spouse to the Community Spouse. In order to get the increase in the MMMNA approved, the Community Spouse must contact the Medicaid caseworker assigned to the nursing home spouse, and apply for the increase based on the new monthly payments.

What this technique really does is use a portion of the nursing home spouse's income to provide extra cash for the Community Spouse, to use for home repairs and improvements, vacations, new car, etc. This is money that otherwise would have been wasted, in that it would have only reduced what the state would otherwise have paid to the nursing home. Of course, it also increases the amount the state may be able to seek via estate recovery following the nursing home spouse's death, but as discussed in this book, it's unlikely the state will ever get that full amount, anyhow.

Family Allowance

An additional amount may be deducted from the nursing home spouse's income before paying the nursing home, if certain other family members are living in the home with the Community Spouse. For these purposes, the term "family member" only includes minor or dependent children, dependent parents, or dependent siblings of the nursing home spouse or of the Community Spouse who are residing with the Community Spouse. To calculate this, you subtract the income of all such family members from the MMMNA and divide by three. This amount will be deducted from the nursing home spouse's income and paid over to the Community Spouse for the benefit of the family member. This payment does not count as part of the MMMNA, however, so it is not subject to the MMMNA cap of $3,853.50.

Support Obligations

Note that countable income is *not* reduced by obligations of support such as that legally owed to an ex-spouse. Thus, if a Medicaid applicant has income over the threshold to qualify for Medicaid in his state, he will not be able to reduce his countable income by the amount of his court-ordered alimony payments.

Fair Hearings

In cases where even the maximum MMMNA is not enough to cover the essential monthly living expenses of the Community Spouse, you can ask for a Fair Hearing before the state Medicaid agency. A Fair Hearing is an administrative appeal within the Medicaid state agency that makes the determination of financial eligibility for Medicaid. It is usually an informal proceeding, but it is a good idea to bring an attorney with you.

For example, the Community Spouse may have unusually high living expenses, very high prescription drug costs, or a dependent relative living with him with expenses that exceed the family allowance. If he is successful at the Fair Hearing, he will be permitted to shift a greater amount of income from the nursing home spouse to himself each month.

The test is whether the Community Spouse needs income above even the maximum MMMNA, "due to exceptional circumstances resulting in significant financial duress."

For example, if the Community Spouse lives in assisted living or at home with full-time home health care, the costs can easily exceed $4,000 per month. In such a case, there is a good argument for an increased MMMNA, and requesting a Fair Hearing would be the way to do this.

Court Order of Support

If the maximum MMMNA is still insufficient to meet the monthly income needs of the Community Spouse, the Community Spouse can petition the local court for an Order of Support. The Order will set forth the amount of income that the nursing home spouse must pay each month to the Community Spouse. This Order must be recognized by the Medicaid agency. The petition to the court should be done prior to applying for Medicaid, but may be done before or after the "resource assessment" (see *Snapshot Rule,* Chapter 7).

Chapter 7

ASSET QUALIFICATION RULES

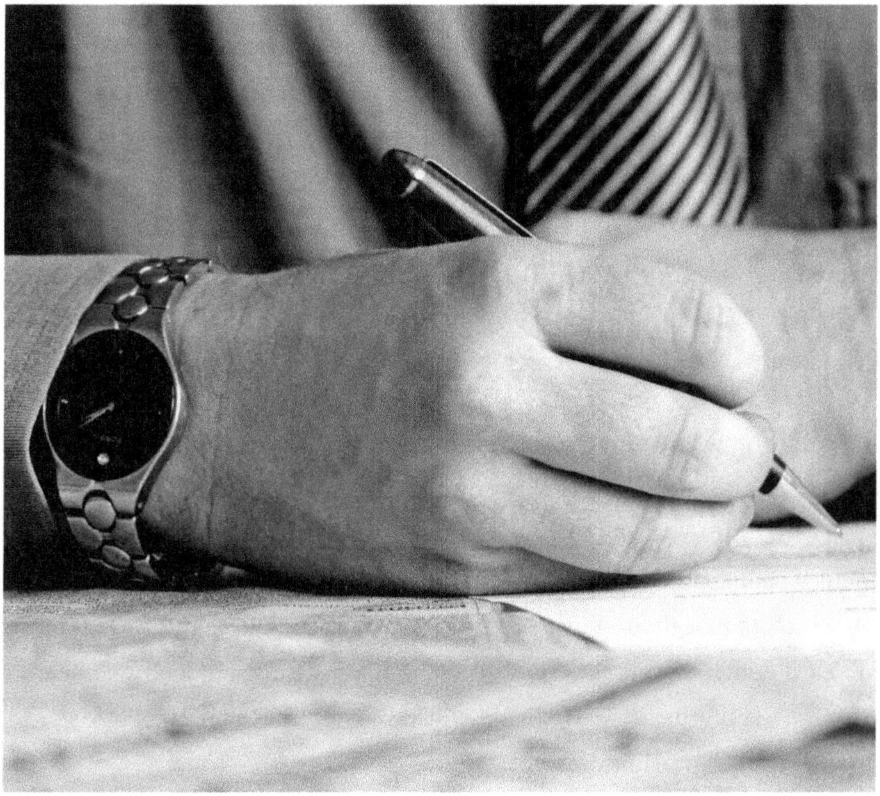

What's Counted, What's Excluded?

Although there are strict limits as to how much money and other assets a person or married couple may have in order to qualify for Medicaid, not all assets will count against the Medicaid applicant. Certain assets are countable, some are deemed unavailable, and others are specifically excluded by statute.

In determining if one spouse of a married couple can qualify for Medicaid, the state Medicaid agency will consider all assets of *both* spouses, whether owned separately or jointly, according to the rules below, and then determine if they are countable, unavailable, or excluded. The Community Spouse will then be allowed to "protect" a certain amount of the countable assets (as more fully explained at *Married*, Chapter 6).

Valuation

In determining what value your various assets have for purposes of Medicaid eligibility, it is your net equity that counts. In other words, an asset's value is the price that it can reasonably be expected to sell for on the open market in the particular geographic area involved, minus any encumbrances (i.e., debt) on the asset. Note that if you have $10,000 in cash in the bank, and $10,000 in credit card debt, the debt will *not* be netted against the cash! You will need to pay off the debt, otherwise Medicaid will simply count that $10,000 toward your asset limit, ignoring the debt.

Countable Assets

If you can spend it or convert it to cash, it is generally countable. Here are the primary examples of "countable" assets:

- Cash, checking and savings accounts
- CDs
- Stocks, bonds, mutual funds

- ④ Joint bank accounts (see discussion under *Joint Account Interests* in Chapter 8)
- ④ IRA, 401(k), 403(b), TIAA-CREF, and other retirement-type accounts (with exceptions discussed below)
- ④ Life insurance cash values (if the total face value of all policies—other than term insurance and burial insurance—exceeds the allowable amount which is $1,500 in most states)
- ④ Annuities not yet in pay status (and many that *are* in pay status)
- ④ All autos beyond the first car
- ④ Trucks, tractors, boats, machinery, livestock
- ④ Buildings and land that are not specifically excluded

Unavailable Assets

Certain types of assets are non-countable, because they are not legally accessible to you:

- ④ an interest in someone's estate, prior to distribution
- ④ a lawsuit you've filed, prior to the judgment
- ④ real estate that cannot be sold because of legal technicalities

Excluded Assets

Certain assets, while still available and accessible to you, are nonetheless considered "excluded" or "exempt," i.e., they will not affect your eligibility for Medicaid.

$2,000 Cash

Regardless of whether you are single or married, if you are successful in qualifying for Medicaid coverage you may retain up to $2,000 in cash or other countable assets. In any month where your assets exceed $2,000, however, you could be disqualified and lose Medicaid coverage. Since that would cause you to lose all nursing home and medical coverage, that would be a very expensive mistake. Accordingly, be careful always to keep the bank account of the

Medicaid recipient well below the $2,000 limit by the last business day of the month!

The Home

General Rule: $713,000 Exclusion. If you are single, and your principal place of residence is a house or condo, it is an excluded asset, so long as your equity interest in the residence does not exceed the state limit (at least $713,000, but this amount can be increased up to $1,071,000 under federal law, *if* the state you are in so chooses; most have not done so). The home *used to be* excluded no matter its value, but that changed with the DRA of 2005.

Note that it is the value of your *equity interest*, not the value of the home itself that is critical. In other words, if you and your brother are equal joint owners of the house you live in, and the home has been appraised at $800,000, your equity interest is only one-half of that, i.e., $400,000, so you are under the limit. Of course, if you were the *sole* owner, then you'd be over the limit. CAUTION: you cannot add your brother's name to your home to reduce your equity value today and qualify for Medicaid tomorrow, because merely adding the name of an individual to your deed is deemed a gift, subject to the lookback and penalty periods. See Chapter 8, *Transferring Assets (Gifts).*

If the value of your equity interest in your home is above the state limit, in order for the home to be excluded you will need to reduce your equity interest. How can you do that? This is covered in Chapter 10.

If the value of your equity interest in your home is under the state limit when you first apply for Medicaid, the home will be an excluded asset. Be aware that if the value of your home has increased above the state limit at the time of your annual redetermination, the home will no longer be excluded and you can lose your Medicaid coverage! Thus, it is extremely important for your family to keep track of the value of your home, and if it looks like it's getting over the state limit, you'll need to implement one of the options discussed in Chapter 10 to reduce your equity interest.

If you are married and your spouse resides in the home, or you have a child (under age 21, or blind or permanently disabled) living in your home, then it is excluded no matter what its value is.

Scope of the Exclusion. Both the dwelling *and* the land underneath it qualify for the home exclusion. You do not need to own the dwelling: you can be living in someone else's trailer on your land, and the land will be excluded under the home exclusion.

The home itself, the land the home sits on, all contiguous land, and related outbuildings (but not a second home) are all covered by the exclusion. (If the adjoining lot is across the street from your house, it still qualifies as being contiguous.) So a house and attached farm can all be excluded. Of course, there is still the $713,000 exclusion limitation (unless one of the exceptions applies: spouse or child—under age 21, or blind or permanently disabled—living in the home).

A mobile home or a houseboat both qualify for the home exclusion.

"Intent to Return." If you have to move out of your home and into a nursing home, the home will continue to be an excluded asset under the rules discussed above, with the same limitations, *if* you have *the intent to return* to your home should you ever become well enough to leave the nursing home. This rule applies no matter how unlikely it is that you'll ever recover to the point where you are able to leave the nursing home. If you are incapacitated to the point where you are unable to communicate your intent to return home, a spouse or dependent relative is permitted to express your intent on your behalf. However, to be on the safe side, it is a good idea for you—as soon as you move out of your home into a nursing home—to sign a statement explicitly stating that if you are ever well enough, your intent is to return to residing in your old home. This can be useful to show to the Medicaid authorities should it become necessary to document your intent to return.

What if you leave your home of many years and move to an assisted living facility and then later into a nursing home? Will the former home still be excluded? No, since the former home is no longer your principal place of residence. Obviously, a short hospital stay in between the transition from your home to a nursing home will not cause you to lose the home exclusion. But any reasonable time where you moved your permanent residence from your old home to a new home, apartment, or assisted living facility, could certainly prevent your former home from being an excluded asset in some states. The key test is if you continued to "intend to return" to your former home. For example, the regulations of some states provide that the home will no longer be excluded if you moved out more than six months before you entered the nursing home. Of course, if your spouse or child (under age 21, or blind or permanently disabled) remains in your old home, it will continue to be excluded regardless of whether you go directly from that home to a nursing home.

"209(b)" States. There are 9 so-called "209(b) states" (named after the federal statute that applies to them) that can opt to use more restrictive criteria than the other states. These states are Connecticut, Hawaii, Illinois, Minnesota, Missouri, New Hampshire, North Dakota, Oklahoma, and Virginia. Such states disregard the individual's intent and instead look to an assessment by a physician or other treatment professional of the likelihood that the institutionalized individual will be discharged to return home. Alternatively, 209(b) states may presume that a permanent change of residence has occurred after an extended period of residence in an institution when there is no reasonable expectation that the recipient will return home, regardless of his or her intent; at least one state imposes this after the recipient has been in the nursing home for at least six months. The result of such a determination is that the house will be treated as a countable asset at such time. (Although not a 209(b) state, New Jersey also requires the home to be sold after the owner has been in a nursing home for 6 months unless the owner can show a reasonable possibility that he or she can actually return home.) Accordingly, if you live in one of these states, you must plan for this possibility: review Chapter 11 on planning ideas to protect the home.

Moving States. A trap for the unwary awaits anyone who moves from their residence in State A to a nursing home in State B and then applies for Medicaid in State B. In order to exempt the home, most states require that you have an intent to return there. However, that negates any claim of residence in State B, necessary to obtain Medicaid, because coverage is based on residency, which requires you to have the intention "to remain there permanently or for an indefinite period." But if you claim the intent to remain in State B, so as to obtain Medicaid there, then you lose the home exemption for the house back in State A by giving up the claim you intend to return *there.* (By the way, there is no minimum residency requirement in a state before a person may apply for Medicaid. For more on this topic, see *Moving from State to State*, Chapter 15.) Notwithstanding the foregoing, some states take a more lenient position, allowing a new resident to exempt the home in the prior state, although others require that the state with the prior home have a reciprocity agreement in place, i.e., the former state must exempt a residence in the state providing the Medicaid coverage, in the reverse situation. Thus, if you are leaving your state and possibly applying for Medicaid in another state, but retaining your residence in the old state, you need to check this rule in the new state. Depending on the rule, you may need to sell your old residence and do further Medicaid planning. And if you still own an out-of-state residence, then you need to know what the rule is in your new state, so you can properly plan for what the state will do should you apply for Medicaid.

Sale of the Home. If you or your spouse sells the home, the proceeds from the sale will continue to be excluded so long as they are reinvested in another excluded home within three months of the sale. Whatever is not re-invested will become countable. Thus, if you are single, those extra proceeds could cause you to lose your Medicaid eligibility. If you are married and on Medicaid, and at the time of sale the house is titled solely in the name of the Community Spouse, the extra proceeds may be safely retained by the Community Spouse and will not cause you (the nursing home spouse) to become ineligible for Medicaid.

That's because of the federal statute that states that the assets of the Community Spouse cannot be deemed available to the nursing home spouse starting with the month after the month in which the nursing home spouse is declared eligible for Medicaid coverage.

One Automobile

One automobile of any value is excluded. Once you go past that first car, additional vehicles may be countable assets, at their fair market value (less any outstanding car loan). See *New Auto, Bigger Auto*, Chapter 10, for some planning ideas related to cars.

Personal Property

Under the federal regulations as amended on March 9, 2005, all household goods (furniture, furnishings, TV, computer, etc.) and personal effects (jewelry, clothing, etc.) are now excluded when determining a person's Medicaid eligibility. This is so regardless of their value. "Household goods" must be items of personal property found in or near a home, that are used on a regular basis, or items needed by the householder for maintenance, use and occupancy of the premises as a home. "Personal effects" are considered items of personal property that ordinarily are worn or carried by the individual, or are articles that otherwise have an intimate relation to the individual. Items with religious or cultural significance are also excluded under these rules. Items held for investment purposes, though, are *not* excluded and their value will be counted: items such as gems, jewelry that is not worn or held for family significance, recently purchased expensive artwork, and other collectibles.

How will the Medicaid workers know whether your household goods, furniture, etc., are normal household items, or if such items are really "held for investment" or "collectibles"? According to the federal regulations, "we will not routinely examine all of an individual's furniture and personal possessions to determine if any pieces are valuable artwork or antiques, [but] we will have the regulatory authority to count such value items as resources when we become aware of such items."

While it is true that your wedding ring and other personal jewelry are excluded, do not run out and purchase expensive jewelry and expect it to be excluded. This was tried in a famous Massachusetts case, where the individual in question, in an attempt to qualify for Medicaid, purchased a $45,000 diamond ring. Unfortunately, the judge ruled that this jewelry item was not excluded but was a countable investment asset. So the moral of the story is, don't get greedy!

Funeral and Burial Funds and Spaces

Bank Account. Depending on your state laws $1,500-3,500 may be placed in a bank account, revocable account, trust or other arrangement, and if it is designated as a burial fund, it will be excluded from your countable assets. However, this exclusion may be reduced by (i) the amount of any irrevocable burial funds such as that described in the next section, and (ii) the face value of any life insurance policy whose cash value is excluded (see *Life Insurance*, Chapter 10). For a married couple, the burial exclusion amount applies to each spouse.

Pre-paid Funeral/Burial. Under federal law, you are permitted to set aside money in an irrevocable pre-paid burial and funeral account established with a funeral home or in an irrevocable trust earmarked only for payment of your funeral and burial expenses (or that of your spouse, if any). Such amount of money will be excluded from your countable assets when you apply for Medicaid. Note that while the federal law does not specify a limit to this amount, many states do just that, to prevent people taking advantage of this "loophole." In Pennsylvania, for example, the limit depends on what county you live in, and the amounts vary from around $10,000 to $19,000.

With a funeral home, the money must either be placed in an escrow account or trust account by the funeral home. Some states require that the contract specifically state that any funds in the account not ultimately used for funeral and burial expenses of you or your spouse, if any, must be paid to the state if you were on Medicaid. In any event, you should not put more into such an account than you believe you will actually need to pay for these expenses;

having any sort of pre-arranged "deal" with the funeral home to pay the excess to your family is clearly illegal.

Life Insurance. Life insurance earmarked for burial expenses of you or your spouse, if any, ("burial insurance"), where the proceeds can only be used for burial expenses, is an excluded asset.

Burial Spaces. Unlike the above-mentioned funeral and burial expense exclusion, which only applies to funds set aside for you and your spouse, if any, the value of burial space *for your entire family* is excluded. For these purposes, your "family" is defined as follows: you, your spouse, your children (of any age), stepchildren, adopted children, brothers, sisters, parents, adoptive parents, and the spouses of any of those persons. "Burial spaces" include burial plots, gravesites, crypts, mausoleums, urns, niches and other customary and traditional repositories for the deceased's bodily remains provided such spaces are owned by the individual or are held for his or her use. Additionally, the term includes vaults, headstones, markers, plaques, or burial containers and arrangements for opening and closing the gravesite for burial of the deceased. Since the value of burial spaces is excluded when you apply for Medicaid, you are permitted to prepay burial space costs without it being deemed a disqualifying transfer.

IRAs

If the Medicaid applicant is unmarried, then in most states the IRA or other retirement asset (such as 401(k), 403(b), etc.) is countable, the same as cash. In a few states if the retirement account is in "pay status" (i.e., the minimum distributions required by IRS rules are already being made) then the balance of the account is exempt, although the distributions would be countable as income to the recipient.

Some states recognize that if the retirement assets were withdrawn to pay bills, there would be a substantial income tax due on the withdrawn amount. Accordingly, those states will reduce the "countable" amount by an estimated amount of the tax, e.g., 20%. If no such reduction is permitted in your state, you may be better off withdrawing the entire amount of the retirement assets and paying the taxes immediately as an estimated tax, since otherwise Medicaid will ignore the amount of taxes you *will* owe on that withdrawal come next year once you file your income tax return, in effect over-valuing your retirement assets by the amount of the tax you'll owe. If the withdrawal will kick you into a higher tax bracket, try to withdraw half this year and half on January 2 of next year; that will divide the taxable distributions between two tax years, possibly saving you some money.

If the Medicaid applicant is married, many states do not count the retirement assets of the Community Spouse. In these states, then, the Community Spouse may retain the $157,994 CSRA *in addition to all of their own retirement assets.* Other states are not so generous and count the retirement assets of both spouses the same as cash in the bank.

Property Used in a Trade or Business

According to federal law, real or personal property "essential to self-support" that is currently used in a trade or business is excluded from resources *regardless of its value* or rate of return.

For example, if you have a working farm, the land, tool sheds, livestock and equipment would all be excluded. A small family-owned business would also qualify under this exclusion. This seems to have little application to an unmarried individual who is in a nursing home, since such person will of course not be able to argue that he or she is currently using such property for self-support. However, for a married couple, it could exclude a significant amount of property so long as it is still in current use by the Community Spouse in a trade or business or as an employee. Unfortunately, many states have ignored this rule or limited it to the $6,000/6% amount discussed below, which should only be applied to *non*-business property.

Non-Business Property Used for Self-Support

If real or personal property is *not* used in a trade or business, only the first $6,000 of value is excluded, *if* it generates at least a 6% return on the amount excluded.

> **Example:**
>
> If you own a separate lot of land worth $10,000, and you rent it out to someone who moved his own mobile home onto the lot, as long as it generates at least $600 of income each year, $6,000 of the land's value may be excluded (the income must be prorated to the entire lot).

Life Insurance

Only the cash value of a life insurance policy owned by the Medicaid applicant is counted; thus, all term life insurance policies are ignored. Also, if the total face value of all life insurance policies—other than term insurance and burial insurance—is less than $1,500, then the cash value is ignored.

If you are applying for Medicaid and already have a term policy in effect, you won't be able to divert any of your income to keep that policy in force, once you are on Medicaid. If your family realizes that your life expectancy is reduced and thus it makes sense not to let the policy lapse, they should consider paying the annual premiums themselves, out of their own pockets. It is also advisable to transfer ownership of the policy to another family member, so that family member will be the one to receive premium notices, etc.

Married

Community Spouse Resource Allowance (CSRA)

The basic rules discussed above as to when an asset is counted, unavailable or excluded apply to married couples and unmarried individuals alike. In either case, the person applying for Medicaid cannot have more than $2,000 in countable assets. However, unlike how *income* is separately counted for each spouse, a married couple's assets are added together when determining the allowable assets each spouse can keep. Thus, it doesn't matter how an asset is titled: husband's name, wife's name, or joint names—it's all treated the same for these purposes. (Note that community property rules and prenuptial and postnuptial agreements are all ignored by Medicaid for these purposes.)

All assets of either spouse are deemed available to the spouse applying for Medicaid, but only to the extent such assets exceed a certain protected amount (in addition to the $2,000 basic exclusion allowed the nursing home spouse).

This "protected amount" is known as the Community Spouse Resource Allowance, or CSRA, and is currently set at a maximum of $157,994 (federal figure, updated annually). All other countable assets owned by the couple, regardless of which spouse owns the asset, must be "spent down," converted into non-countable assets, or otherwise disposed of by the couple, before the nursing home spouse will be eligible for Medicaid. Most states don't care what you do with the excess assets (other than gifting), so long as the countable assets are reduced to the CSRA + $2,000 by the time the couple applies for Medicaid. This is in accord with the language of the federal statute. Regardless, a few states nonetheless insist that the assets in excess of the CSRA must be spent down only on the care of the nursing home spouse. There does not appear to be any support for this position in the federal law.

Let's take a look at how the CSRA is determined.

Fifty Percent States

In 36 states (plus Washington, D.C.), the Community Spouse may protect no more than 50% of the total countable assets of the couple, with a minimum CSRA of $31,598.70 and a maximum CSRA of $157,994 (federal figures, updated annually). Some of these states round up the minimum figure or even set the minimum amount much higher, e.g., $75,000.

However to see if your state is a "50% state," go to https://www.medicaidplanningassistance.org/state-specific-medicaid-eligibility/ and click on your state name. Then click on "Asset Definitions & Exceptions." In the section titled "Treatment of Assets for a Couple", if it says something like "CSRA allows the community spouse (the non-applicant spouse) to retain 50% of the couple's assets…", this indicates that you live in a "50% state." Otherwise, you are in a "100% state."

If you are in a "50% state," you must first add up the total countable assets of both spouses and divide by two. Compare that calculated figure to the numbers shown on the webpage for your state for Minimum and Maximum Community Spouse Resource Allowance. If your calculated figure is less than the Minimum Spouse Community Resource Allowance, then use that Minimum number as your CSRA. If your calculated figure is between the Minimum and Maximum Community Spouse Resource Allowance numbers, then your calculated figure is your CSRA. If your calculated figure is higher than the Maximum Community Spouse Resource Allowance, then that Maximum amount is your CSRA. In other words, the Community Spouse can always protect at least the Minimum Community Spouse Resource Allowance, but never more than the Maximum Community Spouse Resource Allowance.

Example 1:

Joe (at home) and Mary (in the nursing home) have a total of $32,000 in countable assets. Joe can keep the greater of $30,828 or 50% of their combined assets. Since 50% of $32,000 is less than $30,828, Joe gets to keep $30,828, and Mary can keep the balance of their assets—$1,172. Since Mary now has less than $2,000, she can immediately apply for Medicaid without having to spend down any of the couple's assets.

Example 2:

What if Joe and Mary had $150,000? You start by taking 50% of that amount, which is $75,000. Since that's more than $30,828 but less than the maximum permitted amount of $157,994, Joe can keep that $75,000, while Mary is deemed the owner of the other half, i.e., $75,000. Since Mary is only permitted to have $2,000, she would not qualify for Medicaid until her excess assets—$73,000—were disposed of in some way.

Example 3:

What if Joe and Mary had $400,000, instead? Once again, you start by taking 50% of that amount, which is $200,000. But since that exceeds $157,994, Joe is only permitted to protect $157,994. The balance—$45,860 plus Mary's share of $200,000—is deemed to be Mary's. Since Mary is only permitted to have $2,000, she would not qualify for Medicaid until her excess assets—$243,860—were disposed of in some way.

NOTE: If you reside in a "50% state," and the total countable assets of you and your spouse are between $30,828 and $157,994, there is a way where you can *increase* the amount of your countable assets and thereby increase the CSRA. This must be done before one spouse enters the nursing home, because it must be completed before the "snapshot" date. This is explained in detail in *Converting Non-Countable Assets to Countable* (Chapter 10).

"Snapshot" Rule: 50% States

In 50% states, regardless of whether a married nursing home resident applies for Medicaid immediately upon entering the nursing home or some months later, the CSRA is based on the value of the couple's assets as of the date the nursing home spouse first entered the nursing home. To be precise, this "snapshot" is taken on the first day of the month in which the nursing home spouse is in the nursing home (or a patient in the hospital just prior to entering the nursing home, as the case may be) and likely to remain there for a continuous period of at least 30 consecutive days.

Such a "snapshot" is critical in 50% states, because the total value of a couple's assets may well change between the date the ill spouse enters the nursing home and the date they apply for Medicaid.

As a practical matter, when one spouse of a married couple is in a nursing home and it appears that Medicaid assistance may be needed at some point, the Community Spouse should make an appointment with an elder law attorney who can assist the couple with making the appropriate calculations and exploring the available options. Once the attorney has all of the "ducks in a row" the attorney may want to contact a caseworker at the local office of the state department of human services to request a "resource assessment." This is *not* the same as applying for Medicaid, which as a general rule *should not be done* until it is *certain* that the spouse will indeed qualify at such time (or unless you're certain you want a penalty period to start running). (For the consequences of applying for Medicaid too early, see Chapter 4.) The "resource assessment" will establish the total value of a married couple's countable assets as of the "snapshot" date, for purposes of calculating the CSRA. Many couples do not request a resource assessment and instead wait until one of them applies for Medicaid. However, the more time that has passed before the resource assessment is done, the more difficult it can be to recreate the assets owned by the couple on the "snapshot" date as well as what the assets were worth at that time. Hence, it is always better to consult with an elder law attorney and get the resource assessment done as soon as possible after a spouse enters the nursing home.

Valuation Upon Application: 50% States

In general—unless an application is filed at the same time that a spouse first enters the nursing home—a second valuation is made at the time of application. More specifically, upon the date of such later application for Medicaid the state will re-evaluate the couple's countable assets to be sure that the total does not then exceed the previously determined CSRA + $2,000.

Although there is a spenddown amount determined on the snapshot date (i.e., the amount of countable assets that exceeds the CSRA + $2,000), there may well be an increase in the value of the couple's assets between the snapshot date and the application date (due to receipt of insurance proceeds, receipt of gifts or inheritances, asset appreciation, etc.). Accordingly, that increase must also be spent down or converted to non-countable or exempt status by the time of application. **It is not the *spenddown* amount that is fixed at the snapshot date, it is the CSRA that is fixed—and on the application date there cannot be any excess, even if this means that more than the original spenddown amount must actually be spent down.**

Example:

> Maria and Pedro have a total of $150,000 in countable assets on the day Maria enters the nursing home. They live in a 50% state, so Pedro's CSRA is $75,000. Since Maria may keep $2,000 of her own, they are told their spenddown amount is $73,000. Pedro does no Medicaid planning and simply spends down the $73,000 on Maria's nursing home bills before reapplying for Medicaid. Because the couple's income is fairly high, this takes over a year. By then, their assets have appreciated so that even after spending $73,000, Pedro has $82,000 in the bank. However, thinking that he has met the spenddown requirement, he re-applies for Medicaid on his wife's behalf. Unfortunately, the state tells Pedro that since he and his wife still have assets over $77,000 (Pedro's CSRA of $75,000 + Maria's $2,000), he must spend that extra $5,000 and then re-apply once again.

Finally, if between the snapshot date and the application date the CSRA figures are increased to reflect a rise in the Consumer Price Index, then those more recent values must be used when determining how much of the couple's assets can be protected.

Since not every state follows this "second snapshot" procedure, you will need to find out what your own state's rule is. If indeed the *spenddown amount* is fixed as of the snapshot date, then that gives you more breathing room since the Community Spouse can retain not just the originally calculated CSRA but also any increases in their net worth between the snapshot and application dates.

Hundred Percent States

In the other states (with one exception), the Community Spouse may keep 100% of the total countable assets of the couple, *up to* the maximum amount (currently $157,994). Only one valuation is made, and that is at the time of application, whether that is when the ill spouse first enters the nursing home or at some later date. Because in 100% states the CSRA is fixed and not dependent on the value of the couple's assets on the date the ill spouse entered the nursing home, a "snapshot" is not necessary. The only issue in such states is whether or not the total value of the couple's assets exceeds the maximum CSRA number *on the date of Medicaid application.*

Example 1:

Joe (at home) and Mary (in the nursing home) have a total of $25,000. Joe can keep all of the assets, since that is less than $157,994.

Example 2:

Joe and Mary have a total of $80,000. Joe keeps not just $40,000, but the full $80,000, since that is less than $157,994.

Example 3:

If Joe and Mary had $175,000, Joe keeps the first $157,994, and Mary is considered the owner of the balance—$17,006. Since Mary is only permitted to have $2,000, she would not qualify for Medicaid until her excess assets—$17,006—were disposed of in some way.

Increasing the CSRA

Up until now, we have been looking at ways of calculating the default CSRA. If the couple is not satisfied with the state determination of the CSRA, it may be possible to get an increase. There are two ways to do this: apply for a Fair Hearing or obtain a court order of support for the Community Spouse.

Fair Hearing

If the income of the Community Spouse is under the MMMNA, then it is possible to request a Fair Hearing to seek an increase in the CSRA by an amount of assets sufficient to generate the additional income needed to bring the Community Spouse up to the MMMNA level. However, since the DRA's effective date of February 8, 2006, all states must use the "income first" approach in setting the CSRA. That means that the Community Spouse's income must first be increased by shifting income from the nursing home spouse (to the extent possible, up to the MMMNA level), before the CSRA may be increased by this method. As a practical matter, this means that this technique can only apply if the total income of both spouses is under the MMMNA (as adjusted).

Example:

Bart is in the nursing home and his only income is $500/month of Social Security. His wife, Louise, lives in the community and her only income is $1,000/month of Social Security. Under the MMMNA rules discussed above, because Louise's income is less than $2,555/month, Louise will be allowed to keep all of Bart's income. However, that still leaves her short $1,055/month ($2,555 – $1,000 – $500 = $1,055).

Because of this, Louise will be entitled to keep an additional amount of the couple's assets, based on the reasoning that those additional assets will be needed to generate that additional $1,055/month of income. It works like this: if Louise can only expect typically to earn 2% on her money (approximate current national average of 1-year CD rates), then it will take what amount of additional assets to generate that $1055/month ($12,660/yr) shortfall?

The formula to calculate this is:

Y= x * 100/P

Answer= $52,750 (1055 x 100 divided by 2)

Note that the 2% income figure used above is merely an example. Some states set the percentage you must use; others let you argue at the Fair Hearing what an appropriate percent should be, based on an average of local bank savings account or short-term CD rates, etc. (The lower the interest rate allowed, the greater the amount of additional assets the Community Spouse can keep.) Other states require you to obtain estimates of the cost of a single premium lifetime annuity sufficient to generate the income shortfall, and the average of the estimated costs of that annuity is the amount by which you can increase the CSRA (you don't actually have to buy the annuity, however). Thus, the particular rules of your state must be consulted before you go into the Fair Hearing.

Don't forget to account for the income generated by the CSRA itself, when calculating the income shortfall of the Community Spouse. You may want to reduce the income from the CSRA assets by investing in something that generates low or no income, such as zero-coupon bonds. After all, the lower the income from the CSRA assets, the more additional assets can be sheltered by means of this planning technique.

If the Community Spouse were able to increase her MMMNA from the default minimum of $2,555 to the maximum of $3,853.50, that additional $1,298.50/month allowed income would permit the Community Spouse to protect up to an additional $779,100 of assets as part of her CSRA! Here's how the numbers work:

Maximum MMMNA	**$3,853.50**
Default MMMNA	**(2,555)**
Increase/month	**1,298.50**
Increase/year	**15,582**
Amount of assets required to generate $15,582/yr, at 2% interest:	**$779,100**

Court Orders

If the Community Spouse finds that he or she simply cannot make ends meet with the default minimum amounts of income or assets allowed under the Medicaid rules, the Community Spouse should seek a Court Order of Support to increase either or both of these amounts. If an Order is obtained to increase the spouse's allowed income (i.e., the MMMNA), then the next step is to request a Fair Hearing to shift additional assets under the analysis discussed above. It is also possible to obtain a Court Order to increase the CSRA itself. These Orders must be recognized by the Medicaid agency in determining the amount of income or assets the Community Spouse is entitled to keep, while still allowing the nursing home spouse to qualify for Medicaid. The petition to the Court should be done prior to applying for Medicaid, but may be done before or after the "resource assessment."

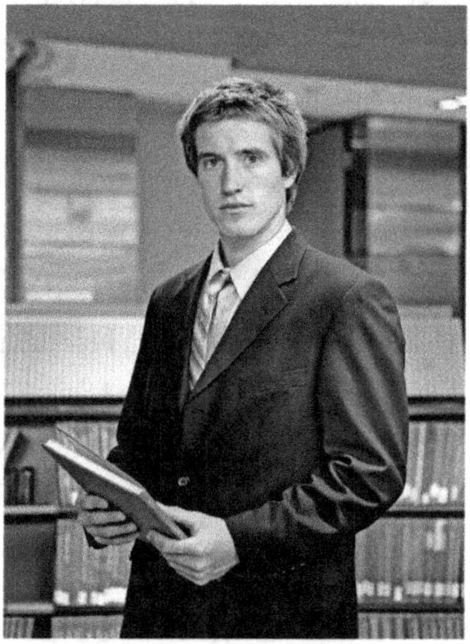

A Court Order may also be sought if additional assets (CSRA) are needed for the support of a "family member" (minor or dependent children, dependent parents, or dependent siblings of the nursing home spouse or of the Community Spouse who are residing with the Community Spouse). For example, an elderly parent or sibling may be residing with the Community Spouse; as a result, a Court Order of support can increase the assets available to cover the costs associated with supporting that family member through a higher CSRA.

Post-Eligibility Changes to the CSRA

Under the federal statute, after the month in which the nursing home spouse is initially determined to be eligible for Medicaid "no resources of the community spouse shall be deemed available to the institutionalized spouse." Thus, even if the Community Spouse's assets double in value because of good investment performance—or if the Community Spouse wins the lottery or receives an inheritance—those additional assets will not affect the nursing home spouse's Medicaid eligibility and need not be contributed toward the nursing home spouse's care. Although annual redeterminations must be made of the nursing home spouse's assets and income, no such annual redeterminations are necessary or permitted of the Community Spouse's assets.

Sale of Community Spouse's Assets

But what if the Community Spouse sells an excluded asset, such as the home? Under the federal statute just mentioned above, so long as the sale is made *after* the nursing home spouse is qualified for Medicaid, it will not affect the nursing home spouse's Medicaid eligibility. The Community Spouse does not have to reinvest the proceeds of the sale; the additional assets are treated just as if the Community Spouse had received an inheritance at that point.

Gift of Community Spouse's Assets

Excluded Assets

If the Community Spouse makes a gift of an excluded asset such as the house to, say, the children, most states will treat this as a disqualifying transfer *as to the nursing home spouse as well as the Community Spouse.* In other words, the gift could cause the nursing home spouse to be disqualified from Medicaid benefits. As discussed below, the penalty period for a gift normally starts to run on the date of the Medicaid application. But here, because the nursing home spouse is already receiving Medicaid benefits, the nursing home spouse would be disqualified as of the first day of the month the gift was made. Of course, since the Community Spouse was the one who actually made the gift, then should the Community Spouse apply for Medicaid for him- or herself within five years of such gift, the gift will be counted and a penalty period will result in determining Medicaid eligibility of the Community Spouse.

Notwithstanding the above, if the gift falls under one of the exceptions discussed in Chapter 14 then no penalty would be imposed.

CSRA Assets

If the Community Spouse makes a gift of an asset that was counted as part of the CSRA, on the other hand, *no penalty* is imposed as to the nursing home spouse, but it is still treated as a potentially penalty-causing gift should the Community Spouse apply for Medicaid for him- or herself within five years of such gift.

What if Both Spouses Are in a Nursing Home?

If both spouses are in a nursing home and both are applying for Medicaid, then there is no CSRA (because there is no Community Spouse) and the total countable assets of both spouses cannot exceed $3,000.

However, if both spouses are in a nursing home at least 30 days and only one of the two spouses will be applying for Medicaid (e.g., one may only be there for a short rehab period), then you can simply transfer all but $2,000 of the couple's assets into the name of the spouse who will not be needing Medicaid. As soon as the transfers have been completed, you can apply for Medicaid on behalf of the other spouse. Because there is no CSRA, *an unlimited amount of assets can be in the name of the non-Medicaid spouse*, and, as usual, there are no penalties for transfers between spouses.

Chapter 8

TRANSFERRING ASSETS (GIFTS)

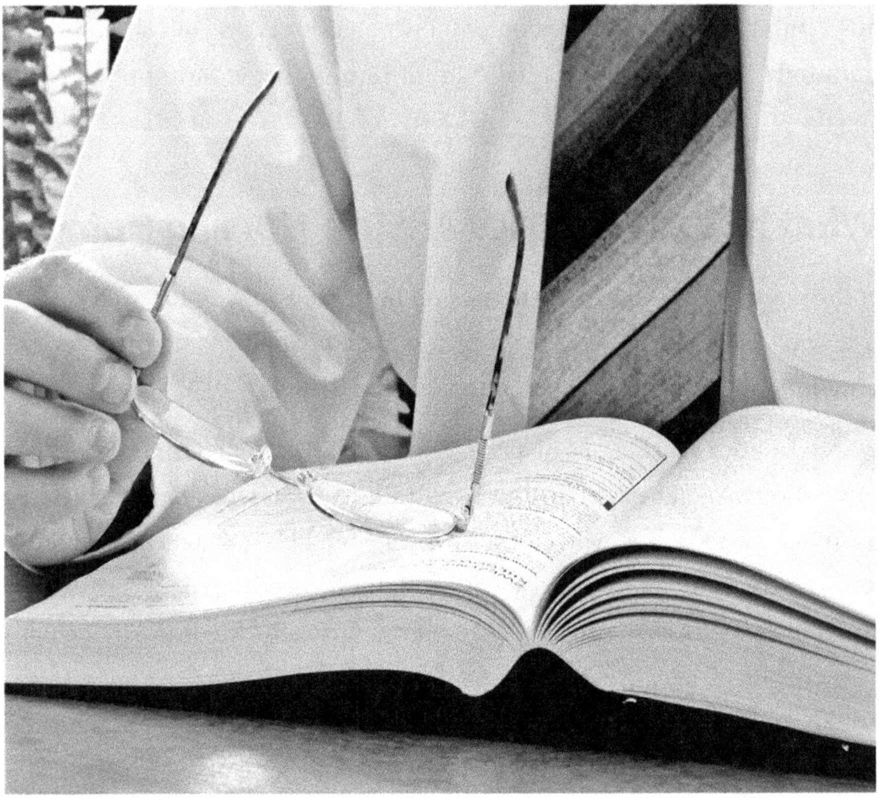

Penalty Period

If you make a gift to anyone other than your spouse, you will be ineligible to receive Medicaid assistance for a certain period of time known as the "penalty period." During this period, even if your assets and income are within the range that would normally allow you to qualify for Medicaid, so long as you are within the penalty period you will be denied Medicaid coverage, barring a hardship exception.

The length of this penalty period depends on the value of your gift. The larger the gift, the longer the penalty period. You calculate this penalty period by taking the value of the gifted assets and dividing that value by the average cost of a nursing home in your state. (Every state publishes this "divisor" figure and typically updates it annually, to adjust for inflation: for the divisor figure for your state, go to https://www.medicaidplanningassistance.org/penalty-period-divisor/ and look for your state.

It makes no difference how many recipients of the gifts there are. Whether the gift is made to one person or ten, the penalty period is figured the same way: it is based on the total amount of all gifts made during the lookback period. (Do not confuse this rule with the federal tax law that exempts $19,000 per gift recipient per year. So for gift tax purposes it does indeed matter whether the gift is made to one person or ten—but not for Medicaid purposes!)

If you are married, the same penalty period applies whether the gift is made by the person who will be applying for Medicaid or that person's spouse. So having your spouse make the gift instead of you makes no difference.

Example:

Let's assume the divisor figure in your state—as determined by your Medicaid department—is $5,000 per month. So if you wrote a check to your daughter for $50,000, you would be ineligible for Medicaid assistance for 10 months: $50,000 gift divided by $5,000 divisor = 10 months.

Now this next point is critical: There is no limit on the length of the penalty period.

For example, if you deeded your $350,000 house to your daughter and son today, and if your state divisor figure were $5,000, the penalty period would be 70 months: $350,000 divided by $5,000 = 70 months. I hear you say, "But I thought there is a five-year limit on the penalty?" Five years refers to the "lookback period" (discussed in the next section), not the penalty period. It is important not to confuse the two concepts. Therefore, you could avoid the 70-month penalty simply by not applying for Medicaid until after the 60th month, at which point the gift will be outside the lookback period. So if you applied for Medicaid in month 61, the gift of the house would be ignored for Medicaid eligibility purposes.

Example:

On March 1, 2019, John transferred his $350,000 house and $25,000 in cash to his three children. How long must he wait to be eligible for Medicaid benefits? If John applied for Medicaid benefits the same day and was otherwise eligible, assuming the state divisor figure is $5,000, John would not be covered for 75 months: total amount of gifts ($350,000 + $25,000 = $375,000) divided by $5,000 = 75 months. And if John applied for Medicaid *at any time before* March 1, 2024, i.e., before the lookback period had expired, he would still be told he was ineligible for Medicaid for another 75 months. Clearly he would be better off not to apply until *at least* after March 1, 2024; at that point, the two gifts will be ignored since they would be outside of the lookback period. **Result:** By waiting until after March 1, 2024 to apply, John's Medicaid coverage could begin as early as March 1, 2024, instead of 15 months later, *easily saving his family $115,000 or more.*

NOTE: Be sure to check with an experienced elder law attorney in your state if you are about to apply for Medicaid after a lookback period. Different states calculate this differently, and it's better to apply slightly too late than a day too early!

Penalty Start Date

As to any gift made by a Medicaid applicant on or after February 8, 2006, the penalty start date is the date the applicant otherwise would have been eligible to receive Medicaid coverage based on an approved application for Medicaid *but for* the imposition of the gift penalty. So if you have not yet made a gift, and your assets exceed $2,000, you are not eligible for Medicaid. If you make one or more gifts within the lookback period that bring you below $2,000, and you then apply for Medicaid, you *would have* qualified for Medicaid *but for the disqualifying gift(s)*, so the penalty start date is the date of your Medicaid application.

NOTE: The state will use the divisor in effect at the time you apply for Medicaid, not the one in effect on the date of the gift. For example, if you make a gift of $50,000 today when the divisor is $5,000, but you apply for Medicaid four years from now, when the divisor has been increased to $5,500, the penalty will be only 9.1 months, not 10 months.

Tacking

What if you make a gift while a penalty period is still running, from an earlier gift you made? The rule is clear: all gifts made within the lookback period are simply added together, and the number of month's penalty period is based on the total of all those gifts.

Example:

On March 1, 2020, you made a gift of $10,000, on May 1, 2020, you made a gift of $15,000, and on April 1, 2024, you made a gift of $20,000. On July 1, 2024, you applied for Medicaid. Since all these gifts were made within the lookback period (i.e., within five years preceding the date you applied for Medicaid), you would face a penalty period based on the total amount of gifts made within this period ($45,000), and the penalty period would start running as of the date you applied for Medicaid. If the state divisor were $5,000, then the penalty period would be nine months, i.e., until April 1, 2025.

Gifts by Married Persons

Under the Medicaid rules for married individuals, a penalty can attach to a gift regardless of which spouse actually made the gift or whose money it was. Because the same gift can affect the Medicaid eligibility of both spouses, it seems like the gift is counted twice, but such is not the case. Assuming one of the spouses applies for Medicaid during the lookback period, the full penalty period applies in determining the eligibility of that first spouse; if the other spouse also applies for Medicaid during the penalty period, then the remaining penalty period is divided equally between the two spouses. Finally, upon the death of one spouse before the expiration of the total number of penalty period months, the total balance will be assigned to the surviving spouse.

Joint Account Interests

The general rule is that joint interests are deemed available to the Medicaid applicant except to the extent that the applicant can prove contribution by the other joint owner(s). So merely adding a child's name to a bank account will not reduce the inclusion of the full value of the account as a countable asset of the parent, for Medicaid eligibility purposes.

In addition, if a joint bank account with a child is set up as an "or" account—meaning either party can withdraw from the account without the consent of the other—there is no transfer until the child withdraws more than the percentage of the account attributable to the contribution of the child. So if, as is common, all the funds in the account were contributed by the parent, then there is no gift by simply adding the child's name to the account (usually done so that the child can access the funds in an emergency). However, if the child withdraws money from the account for his own personal use and benefit, then it is a gift to the child at that time.

However, if the account title is changed to an "and" account—meaning that neither party can withdraw from the account without the consent of the other—then Medicaid rules require that action to be deemed a gift from the parent to the child *of the entire amount in the bank account.* That is because under the Medicaid rules when any action is taken that reduces or eliminates the account owner's ownership or control over the account or any portion thereof, it is deemed a gift of such portion.

Valuing the Gift

The general rule is that the value of a gifted asset is its "fair market value." That means what you could sell it for in a retail sale to the general public in a private party sale.

Automobiles

Look up the Kelley Blue Book value (www.kbb.com). Remember, however, that the one auto is excluded no matter what its value is.

Bank Accounts, CDs

Value is based on the amount you would receive if you liquidated the account. So for a CD, only count the amount of interest already credited to your account.

Life Insurance

Only cash value is counted, so ignore the value of term and group insurance, which have no cash value. Contact the insurance company to obtain a Form 712, which will set forth the current cash value less outstanding loans, if any. That will be the value for Medicaid purposes.

Real Estate

For real estate, you may need to get an appraisal, although often you can rely on the 100% value as stated on your most recent real estate tax bill. This is usually spelled out in your state Medicaid regulations.

Stocks, Bonds, Mutual Funds

Since the values of these assets fluctuate daily, obtain the value as of the date of the gift.

Partial Gifts

Occasionally people get the bright idea that if they "sell" some item they own to their children for, say, a dollar, then the entire transaction is no longer a gift. After all, it was a sale, not a gift, right? Unfortunately, that technique doesn't work. In reality, this transaction will be characterized as a part gift/part sale. The amount of compensation received will be subtracted from the fair market value of the asset that was transferred, to arrive at the value of the gift. So if you sell your house to your daughter for $10,000, and the house was appraised at $200,000, then you have made a gift of $190,000 ($200,000 - $10,000).

Lookback Period

When a person applies for Medicaid, one of the questions on the intake form will be "Have you (or your spouse, if married) made any gifts within the past five years?" (Note that a gift by your spouse counts the same as a gift by you.) What the Medicaid workers are looking for are "uncompensated transfers" or "transfers without fair consideration," i.e., gifts, so that they can impose the proper penalty period (discussed above). If the gift was made too long ago, it must be ignored; it would be as if you never made the gift at all, no matter how large a gift it was. How far back the worker can look to see if you made a gift is known as the "lookback period."

Outright Gifts

When the penalty for gifting was first implemented, the lookback period for outright gifts was 24 months. It was later extended to 30 months, then 36 months and finally to the current period of 60 months. This means that any gift you made more than five years prior to the date you apply for Medicaid must be ignored. For example, if you transfer your million-dollar house to your children but do not apply for Medicaid until 61 months later, then this very large gift must be ignored and will not count against you.

Under the current rules, there is no benefit to making a gift sooner rather than later unless the person who makes the gift can wait at least a full *five years* from the date of the gift before applying for Medicaid. That is because the penalty period does not begin to run until the person who made the gift applies for Medicaid.

Example:

Sally has only $102,000 of countable assets. Thinking she may need to move into a nursing home in a couple of years, Sally makes a gift of $50,000 on January 1 of next year (Year 1) and another $50,000 on January 1 of the year after that (Year 2). On January 1 of Year 4, Sally has to move into a nursing home. By this time she has no countable assets left (other than her personal exclusion of $2,000), so ordinarily she would have qualified for Medicaid. However, since she made gifts within the past five years of her application date, the two $50,000 gifts must be added together and treated as if she made the gifts on the day she applied for Medicaid. So her $100,000 of total gifts will now cause her to be disqualified for a period equal to $100,000 ÷ $5,000 [assuming that's the state penalty divisor figure] = 20 months. If Sally waits until January 1 of Year 6, only the second gift of $50,000 will count against her, since the first gift is now more than five years old. Finally, if Sally instead waits until January 1 of year 7, then she will immediately qualify for Medicaid, because more than five years have passed since the date of her last gift.

Gifts to Trusts

Different rules apply to gifts into and out of revocable and irrevocable trusts. See the discussion in Chapter 9, *Trusts*.

Taxable Gifts

The federal gift tax will rarely be an issue, since it exempts the first $13.99 million of lifetime gifts (2025 amount). However, it is important to note that at time of publishing this book it is projected that this exclusion amount will be reduced to $7 million as of January 1, 2026 when the current law sunsets if no new law is passed by Congress. Some states have imposed a state gift tax law.

To check to see if your state has a state gift tax law go to https://www.wealthspire.com/guides-whitepapers/federal-state-estate-gift-tax/

Note that under federal and state gift tax laws, there is never a gift tax for transfers between spouses.

Chapter 9

TRUSTS

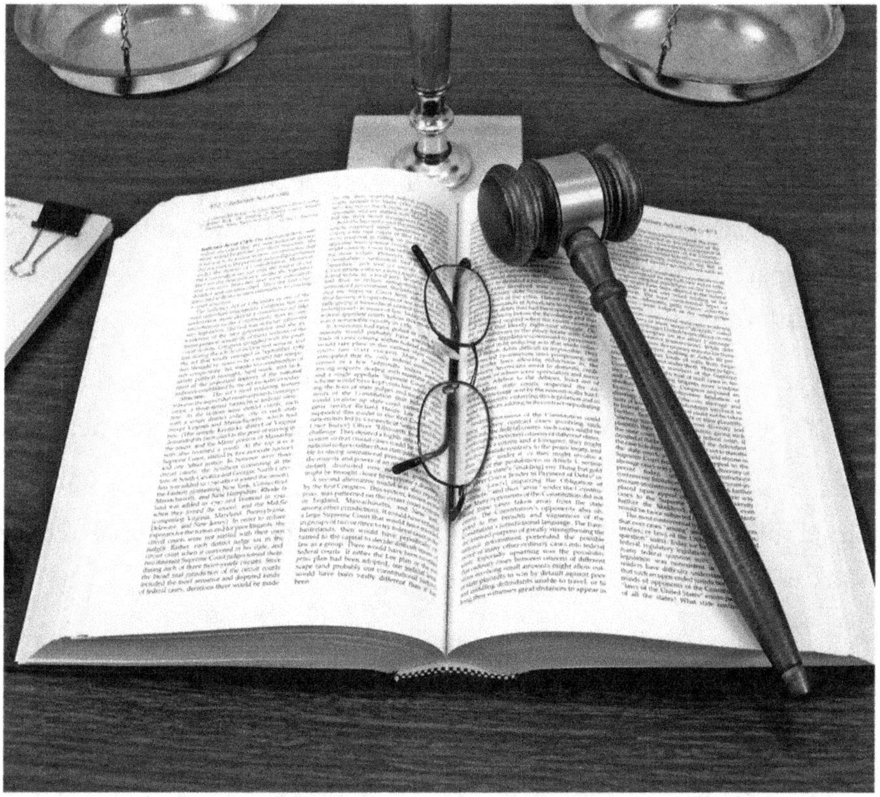

Basic Terms and Concepts

A "trust" is a legal arrangement where one person (called the "trustee") holds and manages property for the benefit of someone else (the "beneficiary"). The terms of the trust document control what the trustee may do with the trust property. It will set forth specific instructions for how the property can be invested as well as who can receive distributions from the trust and under what circumstances.

Trust "property" can be any type of asset that can be titled in the name of a trust, such as cash, CDs, stocks, or real estate. The property in the trust is called the "principal" of the trust. Any interest, dividends or other income generated by the trust property is called the trust "income."

You can actually wear more than one hat: you can be the creator of the trust (called the "grantor" or "settlor" of the trust), the trustee, *and* the beneficiary!

There are two basic types of trusts—revocable and irrevocable—and the Medicaid rules that apply to trusts differ depending on which type you create. Let's take a look at these two types of trusts.

Revocable Trusts

A "revocable" trust is one that can be changed or revoked by the creator of the trust, at any time. A revocable trust is what is commonly referred to as a "living trust." Such trusts are widely promoted in seminars as offering a tremendous number of benefits over a will. However, as a general rule, revocable trusts are not recommended for Medicaid planning purposes.

All Trust Assets Countable

If a Medicaid applicant (or spouse) has the power to revoke a trust, then *all* the assets titled in the name of that trust will be countable for purposes of determining the eligibility of the applicant, other than normally excluded assets (except for the home of an institutionalized individual). Although your home is normally an excluded asset, if the home is deeded into the name of your revocable trust, it loses its exclusion and will now be a countable asset! If this is your situation, you will need to deed the house out of the trust name and put it back into your name (or your spouse's name, if you are married) before you apply for Medicaid. (For the one exception, see *Converting Non-Countable Assets to Countable*, Chapter 10

Transfers To and From

There is never a penalty for transferring assets from your name into the name of your revocable trust. But should you make a distribution from the trust to a beneficiary of the trust, it's treated the same as if you made a gift of those same assets yourself, directly, i.e., in most cases subject to a penalty and the five-year lookback period (see Chapter 8).

Example:

Joe transfers $100,000 into a revocable living trust. He withdraws $5,000 a month later to pay some bills, and a month after that he writes a $20,000 check from the trust to his daughter, to help her with a down payment on a house.

RESULT: There is no penalty period imposed upon Joe's initial transfer of $100,000 into the trust, because he can revoke the trust at any time and get it all back. Also, should he apply for Medicaid, all of the assets in the trust will be countable as his own money, just as if he had not placed them in the name of the trust. This is true regardless of when he established the trust.

The gift to his daughter will be a disqualifying transfer subject to a five-year lookback period. That means that if Joe applies for Medicaid within five years from the date he wrote the check, then assuming the state penalty divisor is $5,000, such gift will cause a four-month penalty period. If he wrote her the check more than five years ago, the gift is outside the lookback period and cannot count against him. If he gave her the check within five years of his applying for Medicaid, the penalty will run from the day he applies for Medicaid (assuming he would have otherwise qualified).

Revocable trusts can be great for estate planning purposes, by avoiding probate, permitting a consolidated management of your assets in the event you become disabled, ensuring privacy of your estate plan, etc. But they are rarely used for Medicaid planning purposes for an *unmarried* individual, for the reasons discussed above. Be careful if anyone suggests to you that a "living trust" can protect you from Medicaid claims and hasten your eligibility—remember that all assets titled in the name of a living trust are countable assets for purposes of Medicaid eligibility.

On the other hand, there can be *some* benefit for a married Medicaid applicant, if the Community Spouse can transfer all of the Community Spouse's assets into a revocable trust and—in some states—eliminate the right of the nursing home spouse to force a distribution from the estate of the Community Spouse should the Community Spouse predecease the nursing home spouse. This will be discussed in greater detail below.

Irrevocable Trusts

An "irrevocable" trust is one that cannot be changed or revoked by the creator of the trust. Irrevocable trusts can be very useful for Medicaid planning purposes.

Transfers To and From

If you transfer an asset into the name of an irrevocable trust, is it considered a gift? The test is whether any portion of the trust may be distributed back to you for any reason under any circumstances. If so, then that portion of the trust is treated as an available asset to you, i.e., the same as if you had put the asset into a revocable trust. If there are *no* circumstances in which the assets you put into the trust can be distributed back to you, then your transferring those assets into the trust is a gift. This would be calculated the same way as a gift to an individual. For example, if you transfer $100,000 into the name of an irrevocable trust and the terms of the trust state that only $10,000 can ever be distributed back to you *if* you had serious medical problems, then (i) $10,000 (i.e., 10%) of the trust is counted as an available asset to you for Medicaid purposes, and (ii) the balance of $90,000 is deemed a gift from you, subject to a penalty and the five-year lookback period.

If the trust states that distributions may be made back to you but also may be made to someone *other than you*, such as your children, then any distribution out of the trust to this other beneficiary is deemed a gift *from* you (and therefore subject to a penalty and the five-year lookback period).

If the trust does not permit distributions of principal back to you under any circumstances, then your transfer of assets to such a trust is a gift, as explained above. In addition, any distributions from such a trust *to someone other than you* are ignored, because the penalty was imposed when you initially transferred the property *into* the trust. They can't penalize you twice for transferring the same property!

If the trust states that the income *or* the principal of the trust can be distributed back to you, any distribution from the trust to you is treated as income to you (for Medicaid purposes; different rules apply for income tax purposes).

If income *can* be distributed to you, in the trustee's discretion, but is withheld for any reason, that income is treated as a resource of yours. If you are already covered by Medicaid, be sure that any such income does not accumulate, possibly putting you over the $2,000 limit. The way to avoid that is for the trust to distribute all such income to you (or to your spouse, if any) so it does not accumulate.

Planning with Irrevocable Trusts

Once your transfer to the trust is considered a gift, it is no longer a countable asset of yours. That is why irrevocable trusts can be excellent long-term planning vehicles: once the lookback period has expired, the trust is ignored. So if you transfer all your assets into the right kind of irrevocable trust and wait out the five-year lookback period, the assets in the name of the trust, no matter their value, will not count against you when you apply for Medicaid. (See *Lookback Period*, Chapter 8).

Example:

For example, assume you are age 65 and believe that you are in pretty good health with little likelihood of needing nursing home care for many years. However, you are concerned that if you did have to go to a nursing home someday, the costs would deplete your estate. Instead, you'd like to leave your estate to your children, if at all possible. Accordingly, you go to your elder law attorney to create an irrevocable trust, and you transfer $300,000 (or a parcel of real estate—even your home) into the trust.

After five years have passed from the date you transferred the money or property into the trust, that transfer will be outside the five-year lookback period and thus cannot affect your Medicaid eligibility. You may even be able to serve as trustee of your own trust (depending on the state rules), so you can continue to manage and control the trust assets for the rest of your life. You can include a provision allowing discretionary distributions to your children and grandchildren out of the trust, giving you the power to make gifts to them at any time in any amount. If it is your home that you put into the trust, you can reserve the right to live in the house for the rest of your life. If you ever need to move, the trustee can always sell the house and purchase another house, or a condo, and if there are extra proceeds from the sale of the house, they would remain as part of the trust, protected from Medicaid claims.

Let's look at a couple of examples showing the effect of transfers to and from irrevocable trusts.

Example 1:

Martha established a revocable trust a few years ago, which is now worth $80,000. Upon thinking about her future, she decides to make the trust irrevocable for asset protection purposes. She retains the right to all the trust income, but in no circumstance may the trustee distribute any of the underlying trust principal to her. On the date she makes the trust irrevocable, she is treated as having made a gift of $80,000 to the other trust beneficiaries. Should Martha apply for Medicaid within five years of that date, she will be faced with a penalty period of $80,000 divided by the state penalty period divisor. So if the divisor is $5,000, then the penalty period will be 16 months. Again, the penalty will not start to run until the day she applies for Medicaid.

Example 2:

Sam creates an irrevocable trust that says that no distributions of trust property can be made back to him unless he is in a nursing home. He transfers $150,000 into the trust. Because there are still some circumstances under which the trust property can be distributed back to him, even though he's not in a nursing home now, this transfer is not considered a gift. A year later, he writes a $10,000 check from the trust to his grandson, as a college graduation gift. The gift to his grandson will be a disqualifying transfer subject to a five-year lookback period. Should Sam apply for Medicaid within five years of that date, then assuming the state penalty divisor is $5,000, such gift will cause a two-month penalty period to run from the day he applies for Medicaid.

(NOTE: It may be possible for Sam to argue that the gift to his grandson was made exclusively for a purpose other than to qualify for Medicaid, which would eliminate the penalty. See Chapter 14).

Income-Only Trusts

What if you needed to receive income from the trust assets to pay your living expenses, but still wanted to insulate the trust assets should you ever need to apply for Medicaid? In that case, what you should consider is an income-only trust. Let's take a look at how that works, now.

If you create an irrevocable trust and retain no rights to receive any distributions from this trust, you are deemed to have made a gift of the entire amount of assets you transferred into the trust. Since you have no access to the trust property, no part of the trust property is countable as an available asset of yours.

But what if your trust document permits the trustee to distribute trust *income* to you? So long as you can only receive the *income*—and the trustee can never distribute any portion of the trust *principal* to you—then the income is countable as your income, under the income rules discussed above, but the principal of the trust is still not countable as your property. So if you set up such a trust and transfer some part or all of your assets into the trust, once the five year lookback period has passed the trust property will be ignored when the Medicaid eligibility department assesses your application.

Example:

Your attorney sets up an irrevocable income-only trust for you. You transfer $50,000 in cash into the trust. You have no right ever to get a distribution of any part of that $50,000, but the trustee does have the authority to distribute the income earned on that $50,000 back to you every quarter.

The full amount transferred into the trust—$50,000—is treated as a gift, just as if you gave it to a child of yours. As such, there is a penalty based on dividing the amount of the gift by your state "penalty divisor" figure. Assume the divisor is $5,000. Thus, $50,000 divided by $5,000 is 10, so that means there is a penalty period of 10 months. If you apply for Medicaid within five years of your transfer to the trust, this penalty period will have to be dealt with. Once the five-year period has passed, however, the gift will be ignored when you apply for Medicaid, and the assets inside the trust, no matter what their value is at that time, will also be ignored.

Dealing with Trust Income

Once you are in a nursing home, if you retained the right to all trust income, your trustee can change investments so as to minimize the amount of income earned by the trust and thus distributable to you. The trustee cannot merely *withhold* part or all of the trust income from you; undistributed but earned trust income will be considered an available resource, possibly causing you to lose your Medicaid coverage! However, reducing income distributions to you is a good idea, because every such distribution must go directly to the nursing home, and once you are on Medicaid such distributions will serve only to reduce the amount that Medicaid would otherwise pay to the nursing home on your behalf. Your care will not change if the nursing home gets more of its fee from the state under the Medicaid program and less from your trust; the nurses or aides on your floor do not know if your bill is paid by you or by Medicaid.

It is also possible to draft the trust so that if you are in the nursing home and no longer require trust income, the trustee can distribute some part or all of the trust principal to your children (for example). This obviously reduces or eliminates trust income distributions to you, and it also eliminates the state's ability to recover against the trust following your death, in those states with an expanded definition of "estate" (see Chapter 16).

Should You Retain Income Payments?

Retention of the right to receive trust income can cause numerous problems, such as the following:

- The income must go to the nursing home once you are in a nursing home (but see prior section regarding ways to minimize income)
- Some states consider the entire trust in which you have retained the income as a countable asset
- Some states may count the income interest under their expanded estate recovery rules following your death
- It can cause the entire trust to be a countable asset under VA Pension rules
- It can increase the size of your "estate" for elective share purposes in certain states, resulting in more of your property passing to your surviving spouse, who may be in a nursing home (See *Elective Share Problem*, Chapter 15.)
- There are other ways to make the trust income taxable to you, even if you don't receive the income

④ There are other ways to get the trust property back to you, such as a "back door" provision permitting distributions to children

Thus, you have to balance the possible disadvantages depending on the rules of your state against the desire to retain all income payments from your trust. Most people prefer retaining the income payments, if it is possible to do so, rather than relying on having to ask their children for money! Be sure to discuss these issues with the attorney drafting your trust, so you feel comfortable with the ultimate decision.

Due-on-Sale Problem

If you transfer your house into an irrevocable trust, you must be aware of the "due-on-sale" clause in almost all mortgages: this states that if you transfer your house during the term of the mortgage loan, the loan will immediately become due in full! Clearly you want to avoid that. Luckily, there is a provision in the federal law that states that if the house being transferred is your residence and it's being transferred into an irrevocable trust in which you are a beneficiary and retain your right to live in the house, then the due-on-sale clause may not be invoked. Thus, it is important that the trust (or a separate occupancy agreement) explicitly state that you have the right to occupy the residence.

Trigger Trust Option

As a way to deal with the "wasted income" problem discussed above, some trust documents state that if you are in a nursing home and receiving Medicaid, no income may be distributed to you. This is called a "trigger trust." Under pre-1993 law, this was permitted, but since then any such provisions in a self-settled irrevocable trust will be ignored for Medicaid qualification purposes. During the period you are entitled to receive the income, even if it is discretionary with the trustee, undistributed but earned trust income will be considered an available resource and will count against you, even if you cannot demand a distribution. And if at some future time after the trust is established, your right to receive the income is terminated, you may be deemed to have made a gift on the termination date (of the present value of your income interest), causing a penalty period. In addition, some states have banned this option as being "against public policy."

Using Two Irrevocable Trusts

If you own a house and are considering using an irrevocable trust to protect your assets, consider the benefits of establishing *two* trusts (these can be two separate trusts or two subtrusts within one trust document).

The first trust will hold only your house and will be a "grantor trust" meaning that all the income will be taxable to you. Of course, since this trust will only hold the house, it won't generate any income. But the advantage of it being classified as a grantor trust is that should the house be sold during your lifetime, the trust can take advantage of the capital gains exclusion normally only available to persons, not trusts. This exclusion enables a person (and a grantor trust) to exclude up to $250,000 in capital gains upon the sale of the house if you are unmarried and up to $500,000 if you are married.

The second trust will hold your assets other than the house, such as cash or other investment assets. It will be set up so that it is *not* a grantor trust, so that if the trust earns income it won't be taxed to you even if you never get a distribution of the income during the year or the trust is written so that you are not an income beneficiary at all (important for VA pension planning).

Should your house be sold and a replacement not purchased, the trustee should be permitted to distribute the proceeds to the other (nongrantor) trust or to terminate the provision that made it a grantor trust (of course, this requires that the trust have been drafted to permit this).

If your income tax situation is such that you pay *no* tax (e.g., you only have Social Security), then there really would be no advantage of this second trust and you can just use a single grantor trust for the house and cash.

Irrevocable Trusts vs. Outright Gifts

What if you have $100,000 of excess assets and must reduce your assets before you can qualify for Medicaid? What if you don't need nursing home care now, but may in, say, five years or more? Should you just give your children the money? Or transfer it into an irrevocable trust?

Here are some advantages of setting up and funding an irrevocable trust, as described above, vs. making the outright gift:

- ④ the trust protects your assets while you are living, both from your children's creditors as well as your own;
- ④ the trust permits you to serve as trustee, with one or more children named as successor trustees, so that you can continue to manage and invest the assets as you see fit, so long as you are able to do so (however, if possible, it is better if you do not act as your own trustee, since some states view that as "controlling" the trust, causing it to be a countable resource);
- ④ the trust assets will not count against you when and if you ever need to apply for Medicaid, should you ever need nursing home care;
- ④ the state cannot go after the trust assets after you die, under their "estate recovery" program, whereby they seek to be repaid for every dollar they spent on you while you were in the nursing home (it is possible that if your state has an expanded estate recovery statute it could try to recover against an income-only trust, so this needs to be checked before you set one up);
- ④ the trust protects the assets from attack by a child's creditors or spouse (should they ever get divorced);
- ④ the trust continues to allow you to control the ultimate disposition of the assets following your death, by retaining what is called a "testamentary limited power of appointment";
- ④ the trust does not increase the Medicaid "lookback period" as compared to an outright gift (this used to be one reason people preferred outright gifts prior to the law being changed in February 2006);
- ④ the trust can permit income to be distributed to you for life;

- ④ income taxes will usually be less, since the income will be taxed to you and not your children;
- ④ if your home is transferred into the trust name, the capital gains exclusion will still be available, should it be sold during your lifetime (not so if it were instead gifted to the children);
- ④ it can permit "back door" distributions to family members should that be necessary down the road; and
- ④ it permits a step-up in basis of gifted assets, saving income taxes for your children.

As you can see, there are many benefits to the trust compared to an outright gift to children. What are the drawbacks?

- ④ A trust costs money to prepare (legal fees for preparing a specialized irrevocable Medicaid trust can be costly);
- ④ it takes time to understand how it works;
- ④ a new, separate bank account will have to be opened up in the name of the trust;
- ④ a federal tax i.d. number may need to be obtained for the trust (although this is now easily done online);
- ④ additional paperwork is involved for trust accounting; and
- ④ a separate income tax return may need to be filed each year (Federal Form (1041).

Self-Settled Trusts

If you are under age 65 and considered disabled, a trust can be established for your benefit with your own assets that will not be counted for Medicaid eligibility purposes. In addition, the transfer of your assets into such a trust will not cause the imposition of a penalty. The trust may be established by you or by a parent, grandparent, legal guardian or a court, on your behalf and for your sole benefit. In order to qualify, the trust must contain a "payback" provision that requires the state to be reimbursed following your death for all the Medicaid payments it made on your behalf during your lifetime.

Because the rules for such a trust are found in the federal statutes at 42 U.S.C. section 1396p(d)(4)(A), it is also known as a "(d)(4)(A)" trust or a 1st Party Special Needs Trust.

Why would you do this? First of all, such a trust can *supplement* what the Medicaid program pays for, improving your lifestyle. For a list of typical items such a "supplemental needs" trust can pay for, see the list at the end of this chapter.

Second, by qualifying for Medicaid coverage, your expenses will be paid for at the reduced "Medicaid reimbursement rate," so even if your assets are ultimately used to reimburse the state, it will leave more of your assets to pass on to your family members (assuming the trust assets are not totally depleted by the reimbursement).

Pooled Trusts

A "pooled trust" is a trust fund set up by a non-profit organization within your state that holds funds of disabled individuals to be used to supplement their living expenses. The contributions of each disabled person are accounted for separately, but the assets of all contributors are invested and managed as a single "pooled" fund, hence the name.

Although it is an irrevocable trust, federal law has carved out an exception for pooled trusts from the normal trust rules discussed above. Accordingly, the transfer of assets *into* the trust is not considered a penalty-causing gift, and the assets *within* the trust are not counted as owned by the disabled person when that person applies for Medicaid. If the potential Medicaid applicant is over age 65, however, some states will treat the transfer into the pooled trust as a disqualifying transfer. Thus, be sure to check your state rules before considering this option!

Because the rules for such a trust are found in the federal statutes at 42 U.S.C. section 1396p(d)(4)(C), it is also known as a "(d)(4)(C)" trust.

The important point is that the contribution of the disabled individual, while excluded for Medicaid purposes, can be used to pay for items that Medicaid does not pay for. For a list of typical items such a "supplemental needs" trust can pay for, see the list at the end of this chapter.

Upon the Contributor's Death

It is important to note that upon the death of the disabled individual who contributed funds to the pooled trust, any remaining funds in that person's separate account must either be retained in the pooled trust for the benefit of other disabled persons or used to pay back the state for any Medicaid outlays it made on behalf of the disabled individual during his or her lifetime. The balance of the account, if any, may then be paid to a named beneficiary (such as a family member) or left in the pooled trust to benefit others. Whether the full amount remaining at the contributor's death must be retained in the pooled trust, or only a certain percentage, depends on your state regulations and the trust documents. You can easily find this out by contacting the administrators of the pooled trust program in your state.

Reasons for Using Pooled Trusts

You might be thinking, if upon your family member's death all the remaining money in your family member's pooled trust account must either go to the state or remain inside the pooled trust, why do it? The reason is that without transferring the excess assets into a pooled trust, your disabled family member may have to spend all of his or her money on nursing home care until it's gone, and therefore have no money for supplemental care. With the pooled trust, the individual would qualify for Medicaid immediately, and yet the assets are still available to be spent for the individual's supplemental care for the remainder of his or her life.

In addition, because a non-profit organization is managing the pooled trust and making appropriate distributions to each beneficiary, there is no need to find an individual or corporate trustee for the disabled individual's funds. Indeed, if the money involved is fairly modest, e.g., $50,000, it would be disproportionately costly to hire a trustee, but the money would still cause the disabled person to be disqualified from government benefits unless something is done with it. Finally, there is satisfaction in knowing that any amount of the trust account that remains at the death of your disabled family member will contribute to the pooled trust's support of other disabled and elderly individuals. Hence, the pooled trust could be the perfect solution; it is certainly a viable option to be considered when doing your Medicaid planning.

Trusts Created by Someone Else

A trust created by someone other than you or your spouse is known as a "third-party-created trust" or simply a "third-party trust." Different rules apply to these kinds of trusts than to a "self-created" trust that you set up for your own benefit. Here are the rules for third-party-created trusts.

If the trustee of a third-party-created trust has an obligation to pay for your "support" or "medical care" or similar terms, then the trust assets will be countable as your assets when you apply for Medicaid. The theory is that the trustee has a legal obligation to pay for your nursing home bills out of the trust property before Medicaid will pay for you. In such a case, all of the trust assets will have to be "spent down" to the level required before you will be eligible for Medicaid coverage.

"Supplemental Needs" Limitations

However, if the trustee is limited in paying for your care such that the trust property can only be used to "supplement" but not "supplant" benefits otherwise available to you, then such a trust generally will not be a countable asset for Medicaid eligibility purposes. The theory is that if the trustee is barred from making distributions that would reduce or replace what Medicaid already pays for, the trust assets are not considered to be "available" to you—and therefore are non-countable—for Medicaid eligibility purposes.

In many states, if the trustee is given broad "sole and absolute discretion" whether or not to distribute anything to you, then the trust assets are not countable for Medicaid purposes. Since you have no legal right to force the trustee to distribute anything to you, the assets cannot be counted as available to you. On the other hand, such a purely discretionary trust is risky because the beneficiary or trustee may move to another state, causing the new state's laws to apply. Indeed, there are cases in several states that have held that the trustee of a purely discretionary trust is required to exercise its discretion to pay for support in some circumstances (causing the trust assets to be countable for Medicaid purposes), and there are arguments that purely discretionary trusts are particularly vulnerable in states that have adopted the Uniform Trust Code. Thus, to be on the safe side, you may want to include the limitations discussed above.

One big difference in such trusts is that they do not need to pay back the state upon the death of the beneficiary for any Medicaid benefits it paid out while the beneficiary was living.

Because these types of trusts state that they are only to "supplement" benefits otherwise available to—or pay for the "special needs" of—a disabled beneficiary, they have become known among attorneys as "supplemental needs trusts" or "special needs trusts."

You'll definitely need the assistance of a skilled elder law attorney if you find that you wish to set up a trust for the benefit of someone other than yourself who is planning on applying for—or who is already receiving—Medicaid or other governmental assistance.

Trusts Created Within a Spouse's Will

Under federal law, if Spouse A creates a trust for the benefit of Spouse B, the trust is nonetheless treated as if created by Spouse B for his or her own benefit. As such, the trust is treated as a self-settled trust, described above, with the result that in most cases all of the trust assets will be considered to be available to Spouse B.

One exception to the above rule is that if a trust is created *within the will* of a deceased spouse for the benefit of the surviving spouse, the trust assets are *not* countable as assets of the surviving spouse, assuming certain requirements are met. Basically, such a trust will be treated as a "third-party-created" trust, described above, and should therefore include supplemental needs language.

Example:

Marsha goes to her attorney to draw up a will for her that leaves all of her assets in a trust for the benefit of her husband, Louis, who is residing in a nursing home. The trust states that distributions can only be made—in the discretion of the trustee—for the supplemental needs of Louis, and no distributions can be made that would reduce any government benefits he would otherwise be entitled to receive. Upon Marsha's death, her assets flow into this trust and are held for the benefit of Louis without causing him to be disqualified from Medicaid. (See, however, *Elective Share Problem,* Chapter 15.)

This type of trust is called by lawyers a "testamentary" trust because it is created within a Last Will and Testament, an old-fashioned expression for a will.

Children-Funded Trust

Following a gift to the children from a parent, the children can make equal contributions of the money the parent gave them into a single trust. One or more children can act as trustee although having an independent (i.e., nonfamily member) trustee will both better insulate the money from creditors of the children and hopefully avoid family squabbles on use of the funds. The trust can name the parent as beneficiary, to cover any of the parent's "supplemental needs" (i.e., expenses *not* paid for by Medicaid, once the parent is eligible). This guarantees that the money will be available for the parent, should he or she ever need it, since it is now out of the children's names completely. Also, if a child is ever sued, divorced, or goes bankrupt, the share of the money the child received from the parent is protected; since the child is not a beneficiary of the trust, it is not a "self-settled" trust open to creditor attachment. The children's descendants can also be discretionary beneficiaries, if the children want to include the ability to distribute to them.

Alternatively, the trust can allow distributions to be made only back to the children, who could then turn around and use it for the parent's benefit, similar to the joint account arrangement discussed below in *Post-Gift Transfers by Children* (Chapter 15). The advantage to this alternative is that it makes it much harder for the state to claim that the trust was "really" established by and for the parent, causing inclusion of the trust property in the parent's countable assets (although this does not offer the creditor protection of the first option).

It is important that the children's funding a trust for the parent is viewed as an independent act of theirs and not as part of a coordinated plan that the parent and the children agreed to in advance of the parent's gifts to them. Otherwise, the state Medicaid authorities can argue that in essence, *the parent* set up the trust *for his or her own benefit*, using the parent's own money, and therefore all the assets in the trust are now countable under the self-funded trust rules. Accordingly, if the children are going to set up such a trust, they should not hire the same attorney who assisted the parent with his or her Medicaid planning. The children should also allow a reasonable amount of time to pass before they create and fund this trust. What's "reasonable"? Unfortunately, there is no hard and fast rule; clearly a week is too soon and five years longer than necessary, so pick somewhere in between! The attorney the children hire is in the best position to advise them about this issue.

Supplemental Needs: List

"Supplemental needs" are those needs of a nursing home resident or other disabled individual that are not covered by Medicaid or Medicare, yet are important in making life better for the individual. Here is only a partial list of such items:

④ supplemental nursing or geriatric care
④ alternative medical therapies
④ physician specialists if not covered by Medicaid
④ dental work not covered by Medicaid, including anesthesia
④ massage sessions
④ haircuts and salon services
④ over-the-counter medications (including vitamins and herbs, etc.)
④ non-food grocery items
④ personal assistance not covered by Medicaid
④ taxi cab rides and other travel expenses to visit family members
④ a specially equipped auto or van
④ furniture, home furnishings
④ clothing
④ cell phone and service costs
④ vacation trips (including a personal assistant to facilitate the trip)
④ entertainment (large TV for the room, etc.)
④ upgrade cost for a private room (Medicaid only pays for a semi-private room)
④ attorney fees

Chapter 10

STRATEGIES TO QUALIFY

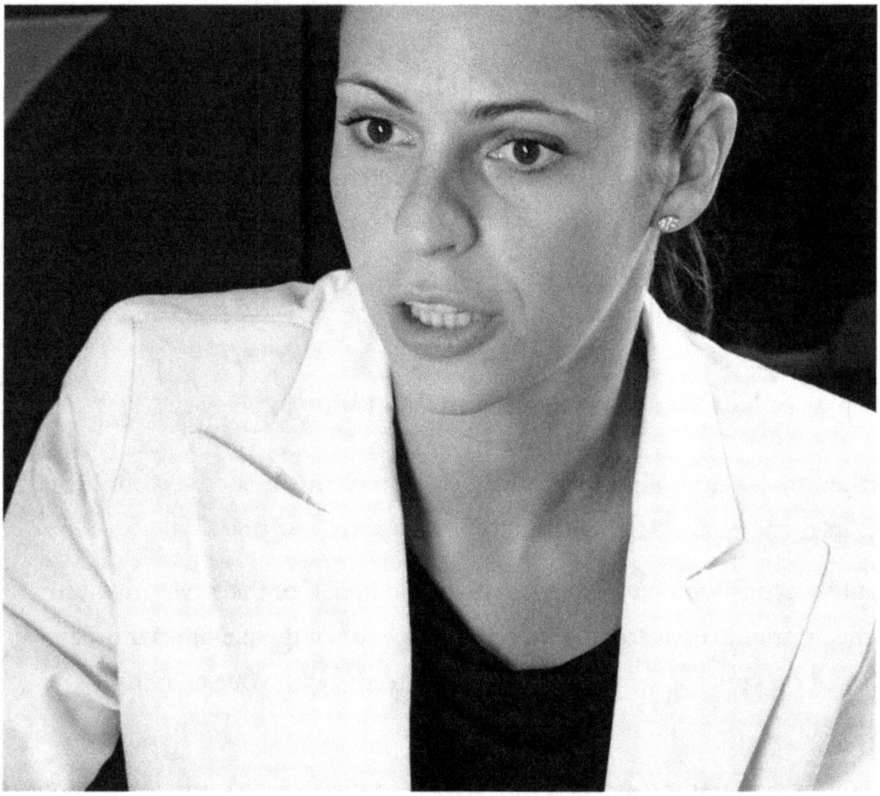

Hiding Assets: Don't Do It!

Good Medicaid planning does not rely on hiding assets or any other illegal means. When you fill out the application to receive Medicaid benefits, "forgetting" to disclose certain assets you own or not disclosing gifts you have made to family members is not a good idea. This is called **Medicaid fraud** and anyone convicted of this:

- ④ is liable to the federal government for damages ranging from two to three times the amount of benefits received wrongfully,
- ④ is liable for penalties of $5,000 to $10,000 for each false claim submitted,
- ④ is liable to the federal government for the costs of bringing the action against such person,
- ④ is subject to a *criminal* penalty of up to one year in prison and a $10,000 fine, and
- ④ may be barred from receiving Medicaid for up to one year.

Further, the state you live in will have its *own* statute related to your illegal act, with its own penalties in addition to those above.

Finally, anyone who files suit against you on behalf of the government for Medicaid fraud is rewarded with a 15-30% "cut" of the penalties ultimately imposed on you, so you better be on good terms with your neighbors and relatives!

As you can see, hiding assets is not to be recommended! With good planning, you will be able to qualify for Medicaid without committing fraud against the government.

Spenddown

"Spend down" is what you do when you have too many resources, i.e., too much money, and you are told that you must "spend down" your assets before you will be eligible for Medicaid coverage. Those excess assets are called your "spenddown" amount.

The classic "spend down" technique is to pay for your nursing home bill out of your own assets until you have reduced your life savings to the point that you qualify for Medicaid coverage of those bills.

In most cases, however, you do not have to spend anything. Instead you can essentially convert an asset that is countable into one that is not countable. The idea is that instead of spending your money on something that Medicaid can ultimately pay for, you pay for something that will benefit you or your family yet not be considered a gift or a countable asset.

There are some very smart ways to spend down. The next section of this book describes these techniques in detail.

Pre-Paying Expenses

While it seems like a good way to reduce one's countable assets, pre-paying expenses such as utility bills, HOA assessments, insurance, etc., will generally not work. Because such payments are refundable (such as if you moved), the Medicaid caseworker will typically insist on counting all those pre-payments as if you never made them. As such, it could cause you to be disqualified from Medicaid based on money you no longer have and may have difficulty retrieving from the entity you paid. On the other hand, paying an entire year's auto insurance or real estate taxes should not generally be a problem.

Converting Countable Assets to Non-Countable

Home Improvements

Since your home is an excluded asset, any improvements you make to your home are also excluded. Assuming you are able to pass your house on to your children following your death, then the money you put into improvements will be money saved. Have you delayed repairing your roof? Finishing your basement? Replacing your out-of-date kitchen? Updating your heating/ air-conditioning system? Paving your driveway? All of these cost thousands of dollars. By investing in your home in these ways, you are sheltering your money while reducing your "Medicaid-countable" assets at the same time.

Adding an addition on to your house is another possibility, especially if this permits a child of yours to move into your house (see *Caretaker Child,* Chapter 14).

New Home, Bigger Home (or More Expensive Smaller Home or Condo)

An alternative to improving your home is to sell your older, smaller home and move into a newer and/or larger home, perhaps one that will allow for a caretaker child to move into as well. Alternatively, the parent may wish to scale down and purchase a smaller but more expensive home, perhaps a condo or townhouse in the city, near the children. Remember, if you are single, that your equity in the home cannot exceed $713,000 (which can be increased to as much as $1,071,000 under federal law, *if* the state you are in so chooses). Under Internal Revenue Code section 121 you are able to sell your home and shelter up to $250,000 of the capital gains ($500,000 if you are married at the time of the sale). You can qualify for this tax-sheltering device every two years. The only rule is that you must have resided in the house as your primary residence for at least two of the previous five years.

Example 1:

Sarah has $250,000 in bank accounts and CDs and lives in a house valued at $250,000. She is getting to the stage where she really needs nursing home level care, but she does not want to move to one, yet. Her daughter, Molly, lives nearby and has expressed her willingness to move in with her mother to care for her. Sarah decides to sell her house and purchase one for $500,000, large enough for Sarah and Molly to live comfortably. Because the $250,000 cash was invested in an excluded residence, it is not a gift and is also no longer a countable asset. After two years, Sarah has to move into a nursing home, and so she deeds the house to her daughter, as a gift. Because of the *Caretaker Child* exception (Chapter 14), there are no Medicaid gift penalties that apply (but there could be *state gift tax* if you live in a state that has a state gift tax). Sarah will no longer have to worry about losing her house following her death, since she has already gotten it out of her name and into her daughter's name, and reduced her countable assets at the same time. Since she has eliminated virtually all of her countable assets, now, Sarah should immediately be able to qualify for Medicaid.

Example 2:

Gus has $150,000 in countable assets and lives in an apartment. Gus's son, Dave, is married and lives in another state. Gus decides to invest his $150,000 in an addition to be built onto Dave's house. Gus then moves into the addition. Gus doesn't worry about whether Dave will "take care of" Gus for at least two years (see the *Caretaker Child* exception Chapter 14) because they created the deed of Gus's interest in the house so that it is jointly owned, with a "right of survivorship" to his son, Dave, and Dave's wife. This guarantees that upon Gus's death, his interest in the house will automatically pass to his son and daughter-in-law. By writing the deed this way, Gus's interest passes outside of his probate estate, which means that most states will not be able to make a claim for "estate recovery" against the son's house following Gus's death. (See further discussion of *Estate Recovery*, Chapter 16).

If you are single, you must live in the community where the new house is located for some reasonable period of time, for this to work. You can't buy a mansion, live there for two days, move into a nursing home, and expect the new house to be an excluded asset! Also, if you are already in the nursing home, it is too late to purchase a larger or more expensive home. The basis for excluding the home is your intent to "return" to your old residence. If you never lived in a house, how can you argue you have the intent to "return" to that house? If you are married, however, it is perfectly allowable for your spouse in the community to purchase and move into a larger or more expensive house.

Example:

Henry and Maude have $200,000 in countable assets and a home worth $150,000. Maude has to move into a nursing home, so Henry sells the old home and purchases a smaller but more expensive home for $250,000. That leaves the couple $100,000, which, in a 100% state, is sheltered by the CSRA of $157,994 allowed to Henry. Maude is now eligible for Medicaid coverage and should apply immediately. (NOTE: In a 50% state, the purchase of the home should be made *after* Maude enters the nursing home and *before* applying for Medicaid, in order to maximize the amount protected by the CSRA.)

Personal Property

Since all personal property is excluded, it makes sense to "upgrade" one's clothes, shoes, sheets, towels, TV set (buy that big-screen TV you've had your eye on), audio components, computer system, musical instruments (buy a $10,000 piano), etc. However, be careful not to get carried away. As discussed previously, spending too much on art objects or jewelry may lead the Medicaid eligibility workers to decide that such purchases are not excluded but are countable investment assets. If so, you haven't lost anything, but you haven't gained anything either: you've taken countable cash and simply moved it into a different form of countable asset, still leaving you with too many assets.

New Auto, Bigger Auto

Under the new regulations discussed in Chapter 7, one automobile— of any value—will be excluded if it is used for your transportation or that of a member of your household. In other words, even if you cannot drive, the auto will be excluded if it is owned by you and used to drive you or a member of your household around. Note that if a family member or hired driver resides outside of your home but uses the auto to provide you *or another household member* with transportation, it will still be excluded. As an example, in one state the county probate court upheld the purchase of a vehicle costing around $40,000 because the facts clearly showed a dutiful son legitimately needed the vehicle to visit his mother daily in the nursing home.

Thus, purchasing a new car or larger car (e.g., one that will accommodate a wheelchair or electric mobility scooter) is a good way to move assets from the countable column to the non-countable column. Oftentimes the older generation has held onto an older vehicle, since they have developed admirable traits of frugality. However, now is the time to sell or trade-in the old model for a new one, since it will enable them to shelter a significant amount of cash. It may make sense to purchase a van that is wheelchair accessible.

Once again, be wary of going out and purchasing a Ferrari or Rolls-Royce: the Medicaid workers may consider that to be an investment, and instead of sheltering the $25,000-$30,000 you might have sheltered had you purchased a more ordinary Toyota or Honda, you wind up sheltering none of your cash! Attorneys have an expression that applies in these cases: "Pigs get fat, but hogs get slaughtered!" So, yes, go ahead and be shrewd, take advantage of every available legal opportunity, but just don't get greedy!

Funeral/Burial Expenses

Pre-pay these expenses (see *Funeral and Burial Funds,* Chapter 7). If you spend down all your assets to qualify for Medicaid, then your family will have to pay for your funeral and burial out of their own pockets. So it makes more sense for you to pre-pay these expenses yourself, out of your own assets. It will reduce your otherwise countable assets and spare your family from having to pay this large expense following your death.

With the average cost of a funeral and burial now hovering around $8,500, this is a good way to spend down your excess funds. If you are married, since you can pay not only for yourself but also for your spouse, this alone can usually protect at least $17,000. If you are willing to prepay for the burial spaces of other family members, you should go ahead and do that also. Once again, this can permit you to pay for something that will benefit your family yet not be considered a gift or a countable asset. Depending on how many of your family members you are willing to prepay this for—and the size of your family—this can easily allow you to protect an additional $10,000 - $20,000 in otherwise countable assets.

Income-Producing Property

If the unlimited exclusion for income-producing property is available in your state this could be one of the best possible strategies to convert countable assets to non-countable. Simply invest the excess cash into rental real estate.

For example, an unmarried individual could have $2,000 in the bank, own his own home, also own a house worth $350,000 that is rented out, and still qualify for Medicaid. Note that the net income generated by the rental property would be countable, so you can reach a point where although the rental property is excluded, it generates so much income that your total income exceeds the full cost of the nursing home. As a result, even though the property is not counted, Medicaid won't be available to you, because your income will equal or exceed the nursing home bill, leaving nothing for Medicaid to pay!

Be sure to check with an attorney in your state to see if income producing property can be titled in a way to avoid probate by using an enhanced life estate deed, trust, or LLC.

Single Premium "No Cash Value" Life Insurance

A number of enterprising insurance companies have recently begun promoting single pay, no cash value, irrevocable, noncancelable, non-assignable, non-amendable life insurance policies. These are issued with no or only minimal medical examinations, and the insured can be as old as age 100.

While there are variations in each company's product, the basic idea is the same: since only the cash value of life insurance is a countable asset then so long as the policy states that there is *no* cash value, the entire value of the policy is non-countable for Medicaid purposes.

At first glance this looks like the purchase of such a life insurance policy would be treated as a gift, resulting in a penalty period. However, a 2007 Michigan lower court ruling gave this technique a stamp of approval, holding that (i) such a policy indeed met all the state law requirements to be considered a legitimate life insurance policy, (ii) since the policy had no cash value it was not a countable asset for Medicaid purposes, and (iii) since the purchaser was the owner of the policy the purchase was not a gift. In short, it worked! However, note that the state has subsequently changed its rules, and it now treats those policies as gifts. Apparently many states are also challenging such a policy on the grounds that it is to be treated as a balloon annuity, in that upon its maturity, it pays back to the annuitant.

Based on the above, anyone considering transferring a large amount of money into such a policy should tread cautiously. Be sure that you can get your money back from the insurance company if it turns out that your state Medicaid department treats the purchase of the policy as a gift, or treats it as a countable asset. It would also be a good idea to have an alternative plan ready in case the purchase of the policy does not work out as you had hoped. (Note that a 2006 amendment to the Delaware Medicaid Regulations requires that such a policy name the state as beneficiary of the insurance proceeds up to the amount of Medicaid benefits paid on behalf of the insured, similar to how annuities are treated. It remains to be seen if other states start adopting this approach.)

Annuities

Certain types of annuities are non-countable for Medicaid eligibility purposes. Because of the importance and complexity of the use of annuities in Medicaid planning, please see the separate detailed discussion of *Annuities* in Chapter 12.

Converting Non-Countable Assets to Countable

There is one situation where you may want to *increase* the amount of your countable assets: if you are a married couple where one spouse is about to enter a nursing home and your state calculates the CSRA using the 50% method (see *Fifty Percent States*, Chapter 7). In such case, in order to maximize the CSRA protection, your goal should be to have total countable assets (owned by husband, wife, or joint) at least equal to twice the CSRA. Currently, the CSRA is $157,994, so your goal should be to have approximately $315,988 in countable assets at the time of the "snapshot" (i.e., the date the first spouse enters the nursing home). (See discussion of the *"Snapshot" Rule*, Chapter 7).

What if you have only $100,000 in countable assets and live in a 50% state? Unless you do something, the Community Spouse will only be able to protect half of that—$50,000—and the nursing home spouse will have to spend down the balance to $2,000, i.e., spend $48,000.

But if you own a house, there are a couple of ways to increase the CSRA.

1. **Borrow Against the House.** At some time before the less well spouse enters the nursing home you borrow against the equity in your house. (This must be done before either spouse has moved into a nursing home, because the countable assets must be increased *before* the "snapshot" date.) This can either be a short-term mortgage, home equity loan, or even a reverse mortgage with a lump sum payment. The additional funds will form part of your countable assets, since cash is not netted against the house debt. Following the snapshot date, the loan can be paid back, leaving the Community Spouse with a higher amount of protected assets (i.e., the CSRA).

2. **Transfer House to a Revocable Trust.** This technique avoids having to apply for a loan (see preceding paragraph), but it does require you to have a revocable trust in place. Thus, it is particularly beneficial when you already have a revocable living trust for estate planning purposes. The house is normally an excluded asset and won't count toward your $315,988 goal. However, if the house is inside a revocable living trust, then it is a countable asset as to the person with the power to revoke the trust. So if you already have a revocable trust, contact your attorney to deed the house into the name of the trust, or have your attorney create a revocable trust specifically for this purpose and then deed the house into the name of the trust. This must be done before either spouse has moved into a nursing home, because the countable assets must be increased before the "snapshot" date.

Example:

John and Alice live in a 50% state and have $100,000 of countable assets and a house owned by John and Alice, jointly, worth $300,000. If Alice enters the nursing home now, John will be able to keep and protect 50% of their countable assets, i.e., $50,000, as the CSRA. Alice can only keep $2,000, so the couple must figure out how to spend down or otherwise deplete the balance of $48,000.

Instead, Alice deeds her interest in their home to John. Since there is no penalty for gifts between spouses, this does not cause any Medicaid problems. Next, John has his lawyer create a revocable trust. Finally, prior to Alice entering the nursing home John deeds the house into the trust for his sole benefit. Since the home is now titled in the name of the trust, it is a countable asset, so their countable assets have just increased to $400,000.

As soon as Alice enters the nursing home, they apply for Medicaid. A "snapshot" of their assets is taken for purposes of calculating the CSRA. The CSRA calculation goes like this: Community Spouse can protect 50% of the couple's countable assets, up to the maximum of $157,994. Fifty percent of $400,000 is $200,000, so John can retain the full $157,994 as the CSRA. Of course, since he only has $100,000 of countable assets other than the house, that's what he will really be protecting.

After the Medicaid application and determination of the CSRA, here's what John and Alice have:

Countable assets	**$400,000**
CSRA exclusion (John)	**(157,994)**
Nursing home spouse exclusion (Alice)	**(2,000)**
Spenddown amount	**$240,006**

But rather than spending down the $240,006, the trustee of the revocable trust (which should be the Community Spouse) simply deeds the house out of the trust back into the name of the Community Spouse (it's a good idea, for estate recovery purposes, to keep the nursing home spouse's name off the house). Once the house is titled again in John's name, it immediately converts back into an excluded asset, leaving him with protected assets of $100,000. Since the snapshot is only done once, the Community Spouse does not have to refigure the CSRA and therefore he can keep his full $100,000 even after this transfer out of the trust.

After the house is deeded out of the trust, here's what John and Alice have:

Excluded value of their home	**-0-**
Countable assets	**$100,000**
CSRA exclusion (John)	**(157,994)**
Spenddown amount	**-0-**

As you can see, this leaves Alice with $-0-, so when she applies for Medicaid, she will immediately qualify. **Result:** John gets to keep not just $50,000, but $100,000, fully doubling his protected assets!

NOTE: This technique is not required in any of the so-called "100% states" (discussed above). These states permit the Community Spouse to protect the full "maximum" CSRA even if the countable assets are less than twice that amount. So there would be no point in trying to increase the countable assets just prior to the "snapshot" date for any couple living in one of these states. Furthermore, it will only make sense to do if the total of the combined countable assets of a couple is greater than the minimum CSRA ($31,598.70) and less than two times the maximum amount (2 x $157,994 = $315,998). So if a couple's countable assets exceed $315,998, then in all states, the Community Spouse will be able to protect the full $157,994. Finally, a few states exempt the residence even when owned by a revocable trust, so in those states this technique is not needed.

Decreasing the Home Equity Amount

If you are single or your spouse does not reside in your home, and you have no child under age 21, blind or permanently disabled, living in your home, the home is only an excluded asset if your equity in it does not exceed $713,000 (or more, if permitted by your state).

If your home is above the state limit, in order for the home to be excluded you will need to reduce your equity interest. How can you do that?

Here are some ways, both good and bad (assume the state has not enacted an increased limit above $713,000):

- **Take Out a Reverse Mortgage:** Taking out a reverse mortgage on the house in order to reduce the equity value of the home is not a good idea: if there is a Community Spouse living in the home, the home is excluded no matter what it is worth, so this is not needed. If there is no Community Spouse, a reverse mortgage cannot be obtained unless you—the owner—live in the house. If you take out a reverse mortgage and then have to move to a nursing home, the mortgage must be paid off within one year of your moving out. That will often force a sale of the house, thereby exposing the entire amount of equity to nursing home costs.
- **Obtain a Home Equity Loan:** If you are in the nursing home, how will you pay back the loan? Once on Medicaid, you will not be permitted to divert income to pay the loan. Thus, this is impractical unless other family members are willing to carry the loan or pay it off, possibly in exchange for an ownership interest in the house. If the equity is just a little over $713,000, then maybe this can be a reasonable option to explore, to make

sure the house is excluded so you can receive (or continue to receive) Medicaid coverage.

④ **Deed a Small Percentage of the House to a Family Member**: Another option is to transfer a small percentage ownership interest in the house to one or more children. Although this will be a gift, the penalty period may be well worth it, if it permits you to qualify for Medicaid. In addition, if you are able to wait five years before applying for Medicaid, then the gift cannot count against you.

> NOTE: Some states ignore the actual wording of the deed and deem a transfer of any percentage to one other person as if you transferred 50%! Thus, you would be deemed to have a made a very large gift, incurring a lengthy penalty. As you can see, deeding an interest in your home (to a child, for example) is not something to be done casually or without complete understanding of the Medicaid rules as well as the other legal consequences of adding someone to your deed.

④ **Borrow Money from a Family Member:** The homeowner could borrow money from a family member in exchange for giving them a security interest in the house, thereby reducing the equity below the $713,000 limit. The borrowed money can then be spent down or gifted back to family members. Be sure to have the debt recorded at the local county real estate recorder's office.

④ **Sell a Percentage or Remainder Interest in Home to Family Member:** The homeowner/parent sells a percentage or remainder interest in the home to his or her son or daughter or other family member. The sale proceeds can then be spent down or gifted back to family members. For sale of a fixed percentage interest in the home, the parent would sell whatever percentage would be needed to reduce the retained equity below $713,000; if possible, the deed should include a right of survivorship clause. For sale of a remainder interest, the older the parent, the greater the percentage of the home's value this will be. Since this is a sale for value, there is no gift penalty. This has the double benefit of reducing the equity of the house (if it is close to or over the $713,000 limit) and providing for a non-probate transfer to the family member upon the parent's death, which would preclude a recoupment claim of the state in those states without an expanded definition of "estate."

④ **Married Couple: Leave Percentage to Children or to Trust for Spouse:** Although a married couple's home is excluded no matter what it is worth—so long as one spouse continues to reside in the home— what happens if the spouse residing in the home dies first, leaving the house to the spouse in the nursing home, if the house is then worth more than the state limit? If the nursing home spouse was already Medicaid-qualified, and the house passes to that spouse, he or she will immediately be disqualified from Medicaid, until the home equity is reduced below the allowable limit. Making a gift of an interest in the home at that point will cause a costly penalty period. In addition, leaving the house to the nursing home spouse will expose it to estate recovery upon that spouse's later death.

The thought may occur to you that the home should bypass the nursing home spouse and instead be left to the children, avoiding this problem entirely. However, it may be necessary to leave a percentage of the house to the nursing home spouse in order to satisfy the "elective share." (See *Elective Share Problem*, Chapter 15)

Thus, a better idea would be for the Community Spouse—in his or her will—to leave to the other spouse a percentage interest in the house equal to the minimum amount necessary to satisfy the "elective share" (taking into consideration any other assets that may be used for that purpose), with the remaining percentage left to the children. (First make sure the Community Spouse is the sole owner of the house, which may involve deeding the nursing home spouse's interest in the house to the Community Spouse.) Since the children will receive their interest under the will, there will be no gift and no penalty period. Meanwhile, the surviving spouse will only own part of the house, and most likely that will be sufficient to reduce the equity owned by the spouse to below the allowable limit.

Even if the Community Spouse's *only* asset is the house, then typically no more than a third or half—depending on the applicable elective share law—will need to be transferred to the nursing home spouse in the Community Spouse's will. On the other hand, if the Community Spouse's other assets are valuable enough, it may be possible to leave *no portion* of the house to the nursing home spouse, which would solve the problem of that spouse winding up owning a house worth more than the exclusion limit.

The Community Spouse's will could also leave the house to the children and the spouse in **joint ownership with right of survivorship** among them all. That means that when one member of that group dies, that person's interest passes automatically to the remaining living members of the group. Note, however, that in most states it is either a requirement that all joint owners take an equal share of the property, or it is a "rebuttable presumption" (meaning that unless the deed says otherwise—which it certainly can—all joint owners take equally). As a result, you may not be able to use this option to give the parent a small percentage of the house: if there is only one child on the deed with the parent, the parent will be deemed to own a one-half interest; if there are two children on the deed with the parent, the parent will be deemed to own a one-third interest, etc. However, unless the house will be sold during the surviving spouse's lifetime, in most cases this will make no difference as long as the spouse's interest in the house, together with any other assets that passed to the spouse, satisfies the elective share. In any event, this option can be quite useful, since it's a reasonable assumption that the nursing home spouse will die before any of the children, so the parent's interest will pass outside of probate (to the children), avoiding estate recovery in those states that do not have an expanded definition of "estate".

If for any reason the homeowners are uncomfortable leaving a portion of their house to their children before both of them are deceased, then an alternative would be for the Community Spouse to leave the same percentage that would have passed to their children instead to a trust for the benefit of the surviving spouse. Such trust should be contained within the terms of the will of the Community Spouse to avoid it counting as an asset of the nursing home spouse. (See *Trusts Created Within a Spouse's Will,* Chapter 9) Such a trust can be written so that it will not be deemed to be "owned" by the surviving spouse, so the same outcome as above will result. Upon the death of the surviving spouse, the trust property (i.e., the house interest) will be distributed as provided in the Community Spouse's will. Typically, this means it will pass to the children at that point.

Avoiding Estate Recovery. Whatever percentage of the house is left to the nursing home spouse will be subject to estate recovery upon that spouse's death. To avoid estate recovery in those states that do not have an expanded definition of "estate," it may be possible to have the Community Spouse's will leave the elective share amount in a trust for the benefit of the nursing home spouse, so that it passes outside of probate upon the nursing home spouse's death. This assumes that under the applicable state laws the elective share portion can be satisfied with an interest in a trust for the surviving spouse; at least some states permit the elective share amount to be satisfied with an income interest or annuity interest, so it should be possible to do this within a trust.

NOTE: If the children's percentage will also be left to them in a trust (as discussed above), then the trust holding the elective share portion will have to be written slightly differently than the trust holding the children's share, but both trusts can simply be subtrusts within the same overall trust document.

Transferring Excluded Assets

As discussed above, certain assets you own are not countable for purposes of determining if you can qualify for Medicaid. These items include the furniture and furnishings in your home, your auto, personal jewelry, etc. Because these items are "excluded," you can transfer any of them without incurring a penalty period. These excluded assets are simply not considered "assets" for purposes of the transfer penalty rules.

Be careful of running out and buying, say, a $350,000 Rolls-Royce, or expensive artwork, antiques or jewelry, and then immediately transferring title to your children. Such items are *not* excluded, because (i) the Rolls was not used for your transportation, and (ii) the artwork, antiques and jewelry were not either personal property found in or near your home, that are used on a regular basis, or items needed by you for maintenance, use and occupancy of your premises as a home. In short, such personal items will be deemed investments and therefore countable.

IRAs

The IRA, 401(k), 403(b), etc., ("retirement plan") assets of the Medicaid applicant (single or married) are counted the same as cash. The plan assets of the Community Spouse may or may not be countable, depending on your state law. However, if the plan assets are countable, it is usually possible to convert the plan assets into a fixed, irrevocable stream of annuity payments, starting immediately, typically by transferring the non-IRA retirement plan assets into an Individual Retirement Annuity under Internal Revenue Code section 408 or 408A. By converting the plan to that of a fixed immediate annuity, the annuity rules discussed in Chapter 12 making the plan assets immediately non-countable. *In addition, the state payback rules do not apply!* (The federal DRA statute carved out an exception to the requirement of naming the state as beneficiary for annuities purchased with proceeds of IRAs (see *Payback to State*, Chapter 12)

Of course, you still have to satisfy the minimum distribution requirements of the Internal Revenue Code, so be sure to set the annuity payments so that the person receiving the payments is certain to receive at least the minimum amount under these rules (found under Internal Revenue Code section 401(a)(9)). If the annuity payments are less than the minimum required amount under these income tax rules, there is a hefty 50% tax on the amount you were supposed to withdraw but didn't, i.e., the shortfall.

Because IRAs and similar retirement plan assets (known as "qualified plan" assets) will be subject to income taxation once the assets are withdrawn or paid to a beneficiary, you should try to take out the money from such a plan over more than one calendar year, if possible, so as to spread the income over two tax years. In most cases, this will save taxes.

Income-Producing Property

Many states completely exclude any property that generates income on a monthly basis. They will count the income, of course, but not the underlying property that generates the income. The term "property" as used in this context means not only real estate but other "tangible" personal property (i.e., something you can put your hands on, like jewelry, furniture, or autos, as opposed to bank account interest, dividends from stocks, bonds, etc.). Although a bank CD generates income, the CD is not considered "property," so this rule will not exclude the CD or other financial accounts.

Example:

Maude has $400,000 in the bank, invested in stocks, bonds, and her savings and checking accounts. Because Maude is single, she is only permitted to retain $2,000 of cash. Her son, using his power of attorney, uses all of Maude's assets to purchase two $200,000 condos, and then rents them out to tenants. He is allowed to pay himself a management fee (or, if he does not want to do this job, he can hire a management company to handle all of the management and administrative work involved in keeping the units rented, calling the plumber on the weekend, etc.). All management fees, assessments, real estate taxes, and utility costs not payable by the tenants may be subtracted from the gross rent. The net rent must be paid to the nursing home. As long as the total net rental income is less than the cost of the nursing home, Medicaid will pick up the difference. The deed is structured so that upon Maude's death it is out of her estate, so as to avoid estate recovery. In states that limit estate recovery to the "probate" estate, the property should be titled in such manner as to pass automatically to a new owner upon the Medicaid applicant's death. So Maude should consider titling the house jointly with her son with "rights of survivorship," so that upon Maude's death it passes automatically to the son, avoiding probate and avoiding the state's ability to recover its Medicaid expenditures. Similar results may be obtained using a Ladybird Deed (Chapter 11), if it is available in Maude's state.

"Just Say No" (Spousal Refusal to Support)

Under the federal Medicaid statutes, if the Community Spouse simply refuses to pay for the nursing home care of the ill spouse, the state cannot consider the assets of the Community Spouse in determining the Medicaid eligibility of the nursing home spouse, if:

- the nursing home spouse has assigned to the state any rights to support from the Community Spouse; or
- the nursing home spouse is unable to execute such an assignment due to a physical or mental disability; or
- the state determines that denial of eligibility would work an "undue hardship."

Example:

Mrs. Smith, who now lives in a nursing home in New York, signs a short document assigning her spousal support rights to the State of New York. At the same time, Mr. Smith signs another short document stating that he refuses to contribute to the support of his wife anymore. As a result, *only the assets of Mrs. Smith* may be counted in determining whether she is eligible for Medicaid. Mr. Smith may have $1 million in the bank, but once these two documents are signed, those assets cannot be considered for Medicaid eligibility purposes.

While certain states (such as Florida, New York, and Ohio) have routinely allowed this procedure, others have not. A 2005 federal court decision held that

Connecticut, which claimed that it did not allow "spousal refusal," *must* follow the federal law and permit this procedure. A 2011 federal District Court in Connecticut essentially reached the same conclusion.

Accordingly, even if your state has not allowed the "Just Say No" procedure in the past, you may want to consider having your attorney bring a lawsuit to enforce it in your state. A lot of money could be at stake, and the cost of the legal work may be money well spent. Based on the clear language of these two cases, you have an extremely good chance of winning!

Personal Services Contract

It may come as a shock to most people to find out that adult children in many states are not legally obligated to care for their elderly parents. In these states while there may be a *moral* obligation for a child to care for those folks who changed his diapers and paid for his college education, there is no legal obligation to do so. However, a few states do have laws on the books that impose a legal obligation on the children to pay for their parents' needs in certain situations (see the discussion under "Filial Responsibility Laws" in Chapter 4).

Regardless of the law in your state, it can be a good way to reduce a parent's countable assets by having a child charge the parent for any caregiving the child performs for the parent. A child or other family member is permitted to contract with the parent to provide personal care to the parent. Such payments will help to deplete the parent's countable assets without causing imposition of a penalty. After all, as long as the payments are reasonable and in line with the going rate for similar services provided by commercial companies in the same general geographic area, the parent is getting fair value for his or her money.

Since all such contracts will be scrutinized by the Medicaid agency in your state, be sure to follow the following guidelines:

- ④ Prepare a written contract prior to the delivery of the personal care services

- ④ Detail what types of services are included and what are excluded (e.g., non-medical care only; cooking meals; light housekeeping; assistance with activities of daily living)
- ④ Have the parent and the person agreeing to perform the services both sign the contract (if the parent is unable to sign due to mental incapacity, have the agent under a durable power of attorney sign on the parent's behalf)
- ④ Have all signatures notarized at the time of signing
- ④ Date the contract
- ④ Make sure that the rate charged is comparable to locally available equivalent commercial rates. Call two or three local elder care companies to get a good idea of what is fair and reasonable for the type of services to be provided under the contract. If the rate charged exceeds the going rate by a significant amount, the Medicaid workers may decide that it's really a hidden gift, and impose a penalty. After all, if your parent can hire a commercial caregiver at $20/hour, and you're charging $50/hour, then the $30/hour rate difference is really a gift to you from your parent.
- ④ Keep an accurate log of all services performed and money received, after the contract is signed. (you'll need that information for income tax purposes).

Life Care Contract

Some states permit a parent to pay a child a lump sum in advance, for life care. Such a "Life Care Contract" is more difficult to prepare and calculate, since the amount and duration of care will depend on the age, health, and needs of the parent, going forward for many years. However, the advantage of such a contract is that it permits the immediate depletion of the parent's countable assets without it being a penalty-causing gift. As such, if this is permitted in your state, it is something you may want to discuss with your elder law attorney.

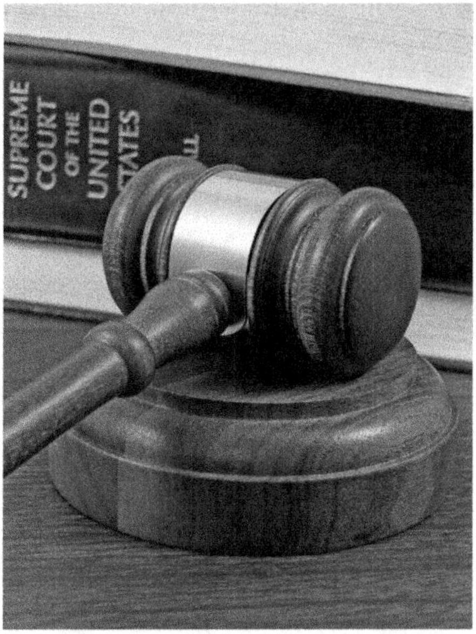

Unfortunately, some states do not recognize such a contract, deeming any money transferred under such a contract to be countable resources or a penalty-causing gift. In the states that recognize such contracts it is important that the Life Care contract be properly written, following the requirements of a personal service contract, and delineate the lump sum fee that is being paid. These contracts must be executed prior to filing a Medicaid application or the state will consider the sum to be a gift.

Types of Services Allowed

In a recent case out of Louisiana, the court held that a lump sum advance payment to a couple's children for personal services had value, even where the parents were already in a nursing home and receiving Medicaid. In this case, the parents' house was sold, and to avoid the proceeds causing the parents to lose their Medicaid coverage, the children entered into a personal services contract with them for a lump sum advance payment. (Note, however, that the same reasoning of this case would apply to an arrangement that is not a life care contract with a lump sum payment.)

The court stated that the children spent many hours performing the following activities:

- prepared the parents' house for sale and arranged for professional inspections
- took care of their parents' regular financial arrangements
- replaced clothing lost in the nursing home's laundry
- provided a phone and phone service for their parents
- obtained several hearing aids for one of their parents
- visited regularly to ensure that their father cooperated with the nursing staff, as he had some mental deterioration
- attended periodic conferences at the nursing home concerning their parents' ongoing care
- made funeral arrangements for their parents at their parents' request
- purchased a record player and radio, found CDs and other music that their parents enjoyed, and ordered cable television
- brought furniture from the old home to the nursing home room and replaced various personal items for their parents
- rode in the nursing home van when their parents were taken to their various medical appointments
- provided holiday gifts
- decorated their room
- brought a pet to visit upon the parents' request
- dealt with Medicaid personnel

Based on all of the above, the court held that the lump sum payment under the personal services contract was *not* a gift, but a payment for services to be rendered. The key to the court's decision was that the services performed under the contract *did not duplicate nursing home services already provided to the parents* and paid for by Medicaid. As you can see, it can be vitally important to keep track of everything the children do for the parent(s) under the personal services contract, as well as how much time it took. Those records may become extremely important should the state challenge the arrangement at some point.

Income Taxes/Reporting Requirements

Any time one person hires another person to do something, and pays them, Uncle Sam is going to want a piece of the money changing hands. Accordingly, if you are going to be paid for caring for a parent, be sure you have checked with your accountant regarding the following issues:

- ④ your status as either an "employee" or an "independent contractor" (Most domestic workers and cleaning people are considered employees, particularly if they only have one employer.)
- ④ Income tax withholding (state and federal)
- ④ Social Security withholding
- ④ Medicare withholding
- ④ FUTA (Federal Unemployment Tax Act) requirements
- ④ State unemployment tax
- ④ Workers' compensation requirements
- ④ IRS Forms W-2, W-3, W-4, 1099-MISC, and Schedule H

If a physician, registered professional nurse, or licensed social worker has examined the parent and determined that they are a "chronically ill individual" in need of "qualified long-term care services" then the costs of such services may be deducted as itemized deductions on the parent's income tax return as "medical expenses." A "chronically ill individual" is someone who has been certified by a health care worker as (i) needing assistance with at least two activities of daily living (eating, toileting, transferring, bathing, dressing, and continence) for a period of at least 90 days due to a loss of functional capacity, or (ii) requiring substantial supervision due to severe mental impairment. In other words, if you are caring for your parent, their payments to you are taxable income to you, but most likely also deductible expenses to them.

Payments for Past Services

It is common for a child to provide for a parent's care, even to pay various expenses of the parent, as the parent's ability to care for him- or herself declines. For example, the child may have let the parent live rent-free in the child's house, paid for additional insurance for the parent, driven the parent to doctor's appointments, and paid for food and clothing for the parent. In addition, the child may have spent countless hours taking care of the parent, responding to emergencies, cooking, cleaning, driving to appointments, making reminder calls, etc., often causing missed work time. Can't those expenses and the value of the time spent be tallied up and used to reduce the excess assets of the parent?

Unfortunately, the general rule is "No," since the child's provision of those benefits to the parent is considered to be made for "love and affection" (or satisfaction of the child's legal obligation, in those states with such a law). Thus, if the parent now transfers money to the child in recognition of all those past expenses and time spent, Medicaid will treat it as a gift, subject to the lookback period and penalty period rules. That is why it is so important to consult with an elder law attorney to have a contract prepared and for the contract to document the services and the amounts to be paid to the child *before* any work is done. Such an agreement, properly structured, will not be treated as a gift but as compensation, and is a good way to reduce the parent's excess assets.

Long-Term Care Partnership Programs

Another way to protect assets is for you to purchase a long-term care policy issued as part of a Long-Term Care Partnership program in your state. Authorized by the DRA, this program is becoming available in more and more states every year.

How It Works. The interested individual must purchase a long-term care policy from one of the participating long-term care insurance companies in their state. The policy must be one that is specifically approved for the LTC

Partnership program. A Partnership-qualified policy provides the purchaser with the right to apply for Medicaid under modified eligibility rules that include a special feature called an "asset disregard." This allows the purchaser to keep assets that would otherwise not be allowed if the purchaser needs to apply, and qualify, for Medicaid in order to receive additional long-term care services. The amount of assets Medicaid will disregard is equal to the amount of the benefits the purchaser actually receives under their Long-Term Care Partnership qualified policy. Since these policies must include inflation protection, the total amount of the benefits received by the insured can be higher than the amount of insurance protection originally purchased. There is no limit to the amount that may be protected in this way, but of course the premiums will increase along with the amount of coverage.

Example:

Let's say Shirley purchases a Partnership-qualified policy with a value of $100,000. Some years later she receives benefits under that policy up to the policy's lifetime maximum coverage (adjusted for inflation) equaling $150,000. Shirley eventually requires more long-term care services, and she applies for Medicaid. If her policy had not been a Partnership-qualified policy, in order to qualify for Medicaid she would be entitled to keep only $2,000 in assets (plus the usual excluded assets). She would have to spend down any assets over and above this amount. However, because she bought a Partnership-qualified policy, if she needs to apply for Medicaid and is deemed otherwise eligible, she can keep that extra $150,000 in assets (plus the $2,000 exemption, etc.): Shirley will qualify for Medicaid immediately, and the state will not be entitled to recover those funds after her death. In short, those "protected" assets will be disregarded by the state for all Medicaid-related purposes.

This is something that you should consider, if (i) it is available in your state, (ii) you are healthy enough to qualify for the LTC insurance, (iii) you can afford the premiums, and (iv) you like the idea of protecting a substantial amount of assets for your children by paying for private insurance coverage (i.e., you, not the government, will be paying to protect those assets for your children).

Unfortunately, figuring out how to pay for nursing home care is all too often made in crisis mode, where the family member is already in a nursing home. Clearly it's too late at that point to qualify the family member for LTC insurance. The only option at that point to protect some of the family member's assets is to utilize the Medicaid planning techniques discussed in this book.

Reciprocity. What happens if a person takes out a policy in State A but winds up in a nursing home in State B? The federal government has been encouraging the states to adopt reciprocal arrangements, but as yet it is not complete. States can either be members of the federal Reciprocity Compact or make arrangements with the other states individually as to reciprocity. In addition, states can "opt out" of reciprocity at any time by giving 60 days' notice to the federal government.

Under current rules, two conditions must be met for a policyholder to be eligible for reciprocity in another state: (1) the policyholder must apply to and qualify under the second state's Medicaid program; and (2) at the time the policyholder applies to the second state's Medicaid program, the original issue state and the second state must be members of the federal Reciprocity Compact or the original issue state must have a separate reciprocity agreement with the second state for the granting of Medicaid asset protection. If after qualifying the policyholder for Medicaid coverage the second state later withdraws from reciprocity with the original state, *the asset disregard must nonetheless be applied to the policyholder* by the second state.

Not only must the applicant to a second state meet that state's own Medicaid eligibility requirements, but the applicant must also meet the second state's Partnership rules. For example, some Partnership states may require Medicaid applicants holding Partnership policies to exhaust all of the benefits under the policy before becoming eligible for Medicaid. Other Partnership states may allow applicants to apply for Medicaid coverage (and receive dollar for dollar asset disregard) even if residual benefits remain in the policy.

While these Partnership programs are a helpful addition to available Medicaid asset protection techniques, at present a person runs the risk of paying thousands of dollars to a company in their current state of residence only to wind up in a nursing home in a state that has not yet implemented the LTC Partnership program or does not have reciprocity with the first state at the time the person moves to the second state and applies for Medicaid. Of course, the policyholder would still have the coverage from the long-term care policy itself, which is really what they were paying for.

It is worth noting that most states have adopted reciprocity in one form or another. But unless both the state in which the policyholder purchases the LTC policy and the state they move to later on have reciprocity with each other at the time of the Medicaid application in the second state—and remember that a state can opt out of reciprocity at any time—the policyholder may be out of luck.

Liquidating Assets

In many of the planning techniques discussed in this book you must either gift assets to another family member or sell the asset and convert it to another type of asset. There may be specific consequences to such gifts or sales you should be aware of, so that you can decide which assets should be liquidated first.

Annuities

If you need to cash out an annuity, there may be penalties if this is done within the first few years of purchase. You need to take a look at the original contract terms. Alternatively, ask the broker or agent who sold you the annuity to find this out.

Real Estate

For Medicaid planning purposes, there are really two categories of real estate, each requiring different treatment. The first applies only to your home— your personal residence. As already discussed, your home is almost always an excluded resource, not affecting your Medicaid eligibility. Accordingly, the only reason to transfer your interest in your home, if you are applying for Medicaid, is so that upon your death, you will not own it, thereby protecting it from estate recovery.

Any other real estate you own will be a countable asset, and in order to qualify for Medicaid if you are unmarried, you will have to sell it and deal with the proceeds, or gift it away. If you are married, the non-home real estate can certainly form part of the CSRA (depending on its value), but that will leave little cash for the Community Spouse, so it usually will have to be sold.

If you decide not to transfer your entire interest in a parcel of real estate, but instead to add the name of an additional owner to your deed (e.g., a child of yours), you need to be aware that some states ignore the real estate ownership rules and apply a different rule for Medicaid eligibility purposes when a person's name is added to a deed.

Another difference between residential and non-residential property is that there is a capital gains tax exclusion that only applies to a sale of the personal residence. Essentially, you can exclude up to $250,000 ($500,000 if married and filing jointly) of capital gains from a sale of your home, if you lived there at least two of the previous five years. If the property you're selling is not your home, you will face a capital gains tax of 15-20% on the difference between what you receive when you sell the property, and what you paid for it (increased by any capital improvements). Be sure to check with your accountant, so you will be prepared for any resulting tax!

CDs

If a bank or broker-issued certificate of deposit ("CD") is one of the assets that is causing you to be disqualified from the Medicaid program, you will have no choice but to either transfer it or cash it in. Although there is typically a penalty if you cash in a CD prior to its maturity date, that cost will be negligible compared to the cost of the nursing home if it causes you to lose Medicaid coverage for another month!

Frequently, however, you do not need to cash in the CD. You may be able to simply transfer the ownership to another family member. Since this is not a "withdrawal" of the funds from the bank or brokerage, there is no penalty imposed. When considering what assets should be transferred as part of a gifting program, consider what CDs you can keep and what should be transferred, and finally what must be cashed out. Be sure to consider the amount of any early withdrawal penalty when calculating your "spenddown."

IRAs

Because IRAs or other tax-deferred retirement plan assets will be taxed upon withdrawal, they should be your last choice of assets to liquidate if you live in a state where IRAs count as available assets. Note that you cannot simply transfer such accounts from one person to another, even to a spouse, without first liquidating the account. If possible, try to arrange it so that you withdraw a portion of the account(s) in one calendar year and the rest in another, so as to minimize the income tax hit.

Questionable Techniques

Family Limited Partnership

A "family limited partnership" ("FLP") is a legal partnership where only family members are the partners. For example, parent and children all invest in owning an apartment building, and a partnership agreement is drawn up indicating what percentage of the profits each partner will be entitled to receive, what rights each partner has in managing the partnership, etc.

Such a legal entity is widely used in business investments, and within the last 15 years or so has also become popular for estate planning purposes as a way of reducing the value of a partner's taxable estate, so as to reduce or eliminate estate taxes.

For Medicaid planning purposes, however, use of a family limited partnership is risky because many states have taken the position that such an investment is simply a way to make gifts to family members. As such, caution is urged before this technique is to be followed.

Self-Canceling Installment Notes ("SCIN")

If a parent lends money to a child, and the child signs a promissory note to repay the loan over time with monthly payments, only the stream of payments is counted—as income—when the parent applies for Medicaid. Assuming the loan cannot be canceled, assigned or sold to someone else, the parent has no rights in the money once it is loaned, so the money that was loaned is no longer a countable asset.

That sounds like a good result, but there is a problem with this arrangement: if the parent dies before the note is fully paid off, the balance due is part of the parent's probate estate and the state could now file a claim against that money for all the Medicaid payments it made on behalf of the parent. (This is discussed more fully at *Estate Recovery,* Chapter 15.)

To avoid having the unpaid balance of the note included in the probate estate of the lender/parent—and therefore subject to estate recovery—attorneys came up with the idea of simply having the note cancel upon the lender's death.

Unfortunately, over the last few years many states have banned the use of a self-canceling installment note, and the Deficit Reduction Act of 2005 put the final nail in the coffin by requiring all promissory notes to prohibit cancellation upon the death of the lender if the lender wants to avoid having the *loan* treated as it were a *gift.*

Chapter 11

THE HOME: PLANNING IDEAS

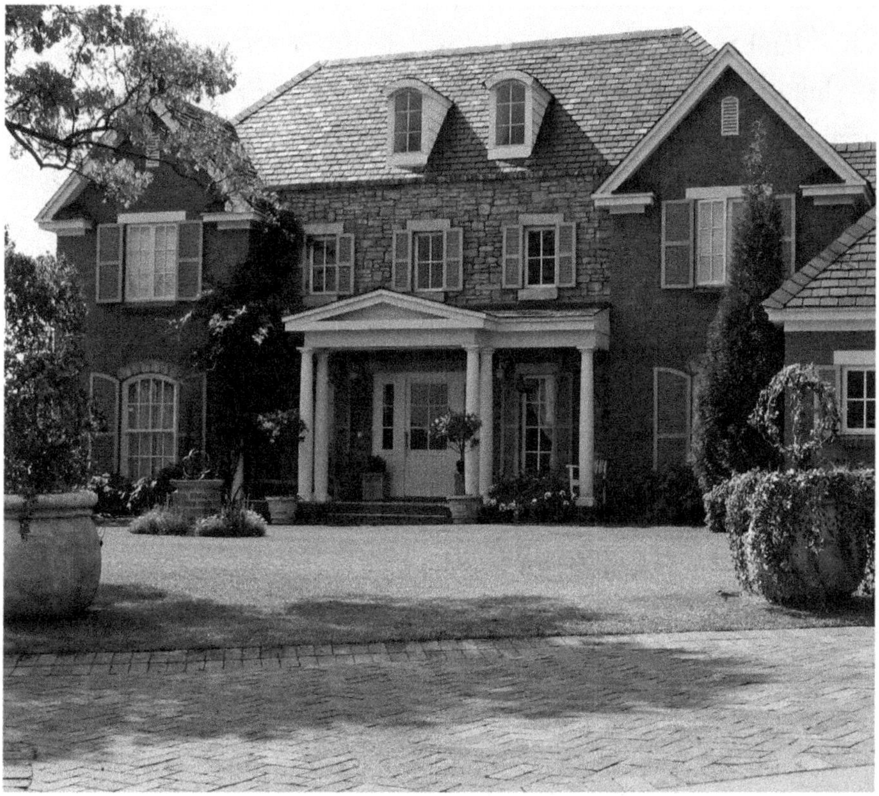

What to Do With the Home: The Goal

For most people, the personal residence is the single largest investment they have. For people considering Medicaid to cover long-term care costs, it is almost always the biggest asset to deal with.

The home occupies a unique position in Medicaid planning not only because of its value, but because it is an excluded asset while the Medicaid recipient is living, but it becomes subject to estate recovery following the recipient's death. Thus, dealing with the home is usually not an issue related to *qualifying* for Medicaid, but rather one of protecting the home against estate recovery following the death of the nursing home resident/Medicaid recipient. (See *Estate Recovery*, Chapter 15.)

> **The goal, therefore, is to make sure that the Medicaid recipient has no interest in the home upon death or at least an interest that cannot be reached by the estate recovery program of your state. How best to do that, and the various consequences of each option, will be the topic of this chapter. (Also review Case Study #2 for an additional discussion of these ideas.)**

Do Nothing

If the parent/Medicaid recipient still owns the house upon entering the nursing home, it is important to remember that the house will not have to be sold to pay nursing home expenses. Unfortunately, some people, afraid that the home will have to be sold, make transfers that are ill-advised or borrow against the house and pay privately for long-term care, when Medicaid could have paid for the care of the homeowner, saving the family thousands of dollars.

Outright Transfer to Children

An obvious option is to deed the home from the parent's name to the child's or children's names. This is a gift for both gift tax and Medicaid eligibility purposes.

Medicaid Gift

As discussed above, a gift to a child is ordinarily a disqualifying transfer for Medicaid eligibility purposes. Take the current state divisor figure for your state and divide it into the amount of the gift to calculate the number of months of the penalty period. To find the divisor figure for your state, go to https://www.medicaidplanningassistance.org/penalty-period-divisor/.

Example:

In 2019, Bobbie Lee deeded her Tennessee house to her son, when it was valued at $350,000. Under Tennessee rules at the time, the state "divisor" was $5,472, so this transfer caused Bobbie Lee a penalty of 64 months! To avoid this penalty, Bobbie Lee must wait at least five years from the date of the deed before applying for Medicaid.

In addition to the gift tax and Medicaid penalty issues, deeding the house to one or more children means that you no longer own your own house. Your children can boot you out at any time! Now of course that's unlikely, but the fact remains that if a child is sued or divorced or goes bankrupt, "your" house— which is now really your *child's* house—can be subject to a forced sale to satisfy the creditor or divorcing spouse, leaving you out on the street. There is also the issue of possible capital gains taxes owing by the children when they sell the property (see *Income Tax Basis of the Home* later in this chapter). So while this technique may work in certain family situations, just be sure you know the risks and costs and go into it with your eyes open.

Add Child's Name to Deed

A gift of real estate is accomplished by signing a deed of the property into the name of the new owner. That seems self-evident, and anyone who has ever bought a house is familiar with how property is transferred. However, it is not generally understood that merely *adding* a person's name to your own, on a deed, is also a gift. Attorneys are always amazed at the number of times clients tell them something like, *"We added our son's name to the deed, so that we can avoid probate on our deaths."* If the attorney asks the client if he or she filed a gift tax return, the client will be incredulous: *"Gift tax return? For what?"*

So let me set the record straight: When you add a person's name to a deed, you have made a gift to that person, equal to 50% of the fair market value of the property on the date the deed was signed. Why is that? Because once you sign the deed, the individual whose name you added to the deed is a joint owner of that property with you, and can immediately sell or give away their half of the property, or petition the court to "partition" (i.e., divide) the property, separating out their half.

There is a presumption that if no percentage ownership is set forth in the deed, all listed co-owners own the real estate equally. If you wish to make a gift of a smaller percentage interest in the property, then you must spell that out in the deed: "I hereby transfer to John Smith of Yorkville, NY, a five percent (5%) undivided interest in the following property: (etc.)" In this case, your ownership interest dropped from 100% to 95%, and you made a gift of 5% to John Smith.

Adding the name of one or more of your children to your deed can also prevent estate recovery against your house following your death if (i) your state does not have an expanded definition of "estate" that includes joint property (see Chapter 16) and (ii) the deed titles all owners as "joint tenants with right of survivorship" (sometimes abbreviated as "JTWROS").

The consequences of adding one or more children to a deed are the following:

Gift Value

In many states, if you are the sole owner of your house, adding one child's name to the deed is deemed a gift of 1/2 the value of the house; adding two children is deemed a gift of 2/3 of the value of the house; etc. However, in some states that is merely a presumption that applies unless the deed language states otherwise. If that is the case in your state, you can deed a tiny percentage (e.g., 1%) to one or more children, and still attach the right of survivorship to accomplish your goals without incurring a large gift. (Your attorney may have to research this, as this is a new concept for many attorneys.) The advantages of reducing the size of the gift are threefold: (i) it reduces the penalty period should you need to apply for Medicaid within the lookback period after making the gift; (ii) it reduces the amount of gift tax that may apply; and (iii) it minimizes the percent of your house that would be subject to your child's creditors.

Exposure to Child's Creditors

Once a child is on the deed, the child's interest in your house is an asset of the child's, and therefore subject to attachment and forced sale should the child be sued or divorced or go bankrupt. Unless you can make a transfer of a tiny percentage as discussed above, your ability to remain in the house may be jeopardized if you add one or more children to the deed.

Loss of Control

Once you add children to the deed, you cannot sell or refinance the house without the signature of all the owners, i.e., you would need to obtain the signatures of all the children. Worse, what if one of the children predeceased you? Then you'd need to figure out who the successor in interest to the deceased child is—it could be the deceased child's spouse or a bunch of minor grandchildren, etc.

Transfer to Children, Keep Life Estate

An alternative method of getting the house out of your name at death, but still keeping it in your name during life so you continue to control it and can't be forced out by a creditor of your child, is to keep a life estate in the house. What this means is that you transfer the house to one or more children but retain a "life estate," i.e., the right to possess the property during your lifetime. Upon your death, the title to the house passes automatically to the child or children to whom you deeded the house before; no additional deed is needed at that time. This can also be described as giving only a "remainder interest" in the house to your children.

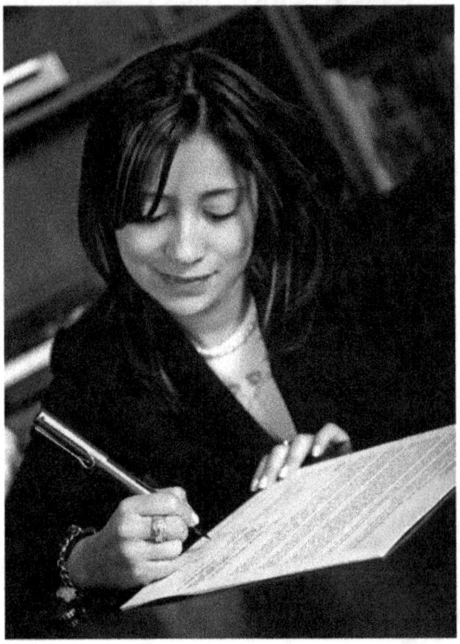

Why would you want to do this? Since you are retaining an interest in the house, you have not given away 100% of the value of the house. After all, you still have the right to live in the house for the rest of your life, and that right has a value you did not give away. So, one reason you may want to consider a transfer of your home with a retained life estate is to reduce the amount of the gift as compared to an outright gift of the house to your children. The gift amount is reduced both for gift tax purposes and for Medicaid eligibility purposes. The other reason to transfer only a remainder interest is so that you can never be evicted from your own home. The interest of your children does not "vest" (i.e., they have no right to possession) until your death. So even if a child were sued or divorced or goes bankrupt during your lifetime, your interest in the house is protected.

How to Calculate the Gift

In order to calculate the amount of the gift you're making to the children when you sign a life estate deed, you first need two figures: your age and the value of your house. Next, look at the "**Life estate table (unisex)**" found at https://secure.ssa.gov/poms.nsf/lnx/0501140120 or in the Appendix of this book and find the "Remainder" number that corresponds to your age. Multiply that number by the value of your house to come up with the amount of the gift. (If you and your spouse both own the house and make a gift of the remainder interest to your children—retaining a *joint* life estate—the value of the gift will be reduced even more. You would need to consult a "joint life estate" table to value your retained interest. The example below assumes a gift by a single homeowner.)

Example:

Assume you are age 65 and you sign a deed transferring your $250,000 house to your children, *but keeping a life estate interest in the house*. You consult the Table and see two figures to the right of age 65: .6797 and .3203. The first figure represents the value of your life estate (as a percentage of the value of 100% of the house) and the second figure represents the value of your gift of the remainder interest (again, equal to a percentage of the entire house). So in this case the remainder would be .3203, meaning that the gift to your children would be 32.03% of the current value of your house. If the house is worth $250,000 today, then signing a life estate deed would cause an immediate gift of $80,075 (32.03% x $250,000). Depending on the state you live in, that could cause a Medicaid penalty period of less than two years vs. more than five years had you transferred the entire value of the house to your children, instead.

Joint Interest vs. Remainder Interest Gift

Once you reach age 77, the gift of a remainder interest will exceed 50%, and the percentage increases as you get older. On the other hand, giving one child a joint interest on a deed will always be exactly 50% (in a state that does not permit deeding small percentages to a child with a right of survivorship). Thus, in such a state, adding a child to the deed will always result in a *smaller gift* than transferring a remainder interest, if you are age 77 or older.

That being said, you should also consider the creditor issues discussed above, which are avoided with a transfer of a remainder interest. Of course, if you plan to wait out the lookback period in any event, then the size of the gift is irrelevant (other than for gift tax purposes, which rarely applies to Medicaid applicants.

Finally, the value of a life estate decreases with each passing year as the person on whose life the value is based (the "life tenant") gets older, whereas a fixed percentage interest in a house will never decrease in value (unless the value of the entire house decreases). This could be important if your state expands its definition of "estate" for estate recovery purposes to include the value of the life estate at the time of the Medicaid recipient's death (see Chapter 16). Once the owner of a 50% joint interest reaches age 77, the value of that joint interest will always be higher than that of a life estate, which continues to decrease as the life tenant ages.

Transfer to Trust, Keep Life Estate

An alternative to deeding a remainder interest to one or more children is that of deeding a remainder interest to a trust. Such a trust must be irrevocable and unamendable in order for this to work. Using a revocable living trust will not work, here, because the remainder interest owned by such a trust may still be considered owned by you when you apply for Medicaid.

The same gift calculations described above apply in this case, too. The biggest differences are (i) if you need to sell or refinance the property, only the trustee needs to sign the deed, and you won't have to get the signatures of your children first, and (ii) you can retain the ability to change the ultimate distribution of the house following your death, should you so desire (through exercise of a "power of appointment" clause included in the trust document).

Upon your death, the interest in your house will pass automatically to the trust, where it will be distributed as you have set forth in the trust document (or as you may have revised it by exercising your "power of appointment" given to you in the trust document).

Outright Transfer to Trust

You can also transfer the entire title to your house to an irrevocable trust. This will cause a period of disqualification based on the full value of the house on the date you sign the deed. Depending on the home's value and a resulting lengthy penalty period, this technique may require you to wait at least five years before applying for Medicaid. However, a clear advantage of this technique is that you will have absolutely no legal interest in the home at your death, thereby eliminating the possibility of estate recovery completely. Also, if you ever need to sell or refinance the property, only the trustee needs to sign the deed, and you would not need to obtain your children's signatures.

Finally, if you ever need or want to sell your house and it's in the trust, this won't cause any problems: the proceeds will just remain in the trust. However, if you had retained a life estate interest in your house instead of transferring it entirely to the trust, then part of the proceeds *must* be paid over to you, based on the value of your life interest at that time. If you were in a nursing home, that could cause you to become disqualified for some period of time.

NOTE: Although you are transferring the entire value of the house, the trust can be drafted so there will be no gift tax. Also, if the house ever needs to be sold, it would still qualify for the $250,000 capital gains tax exclusion, assuming the trust is drafted correctly.

Ladybird Deed

In a number of states it is possible for you to transfer the home to someone else, typically your children, while retaining a life estate with the legal right to sell or otherwise dispose of the house during your lifetime. This avoids probate of your house at your death (and therefore avoids estate recovery, too, assuming the state does not have an expanded definition of "estate"). If you never sell or otherwise dispose of the house during your lifetime, then at your death ownership passes automatically to the individuals you deeded the house to, by operation of law, regardless of what your will says. Because you retain the power to sell or dispose of the house, signing the deed is not a gift; after all, you can essentially revoke the transfer at any time simply by signing a new deed transferring the house to someone else! This is quite similar in concept to a "beneficiary deed," which also allows you to list who will take title to your house if you still own it at the time of your death.

If this technique is available in your state, be sure to consider this opportunity!

Purchase Life Estate in Child's Home

If it is possible for the parent to move into a child's home, this can be a wonderful method of protecting the parent's assets. The parent would sell his or her home and move in with the child. The child signs a deed transferring a percentage interest in the child's home equal to the value of the parent's life estate to the parent, and the parent transfers cash to the child in an amount equal to the value of that interest. *The parent must live in the child's house for at least one year after the deed is signed,* otherwise the Medicaid rules say that the purchase of the interest will be deemed to be a gift to the child of 100% of the amount the parent invested in the child's house.

In order for this technique to work, the parent must be able to prove that he or she actually lived in the child's house for at least a full year after the purchase of the life estate. For example, in a recent case the mother had her mail forwarded to the new address but never changed her driver's license address, tax return address, or election records. Thirteen months after she purchased the life estate she entered a nursing home and later applied for Medicaid. The state Medicaid department denied the exclusion of the life estate and treated the purchase as a gift to the child. Because the parent could not prove she actually lived in the child's house for at least a year after the purchase—forwarding the mail was clearly insufficient in light of the other non-updates to her address—the court agreed with the state that the purchase of the life estate must be treated as a gift to the child. The court also noted that the parent did not have a telephone or utility bill in her name at the child's house. LESSON LEARNED: If the parent is going to do this, be sure they understand the "at least one year" rule and that they make appropriate and immediate changes to their address of record at least for their mail, driver's license, tax return, telephone, and utility bills. It is not enough for the parent to live in the child's house; the parent must be able to *prove* they lived in the child's house for at least one year after the life estate purchase.

Example:

Justin and his wife, Janice, recently purchased a home in an upscale part of town for $600,000. Janice's mom, Eunice, age 76, has been in declining health, needing assistance during the day. The value of her home and life savings together total $310,000. So Eunice sells her home and moves in with Justin and Janice, writing them a check for $302,646 in exchange for a life estate in their home. How did they come up with that amount? Based on the "**Life Estate Table (unisex)**" (see table in the Appendix), a person age 76 has a life estate valued at 50.441% and a remainder interest valued at 49.559%. Multiplying the value of the home ($600,000) by the value of Eunice's life estate (50.441%) gives you the value of the interest that Eunice is purchasing: $302,646.

If after a year Eunice has to move into a nursing home, her interest in her daughter's house will not be counted, since it is considered an interest in a personal residence, and such interest is almost always an excluded asset. Upon Eunice's death, her interest simply expires, leaving Justin and Janice once again as 100% owners of their home. Thus, there is nothing in Eunice's estate for the state Medicaid recovery unit to go after (assuming her state does not have an expanded definition of "estate"—see Chapter 16).

Purchase Joint Interest in Child's Home

Because the life estate interest is fixed in percentage, it can sometimes be more advantageous for a parent to purchase a joint interest in a child's home and then move in, compared to purchasing a life estate in the child's home.

Example:

Assume that Eunice (from the previous example) instead has $400,000 of assets and wants to move in with her daughter and son-in-law, Janice and Justin. If she purchases a life estate, as we saw, the most she can shelter is approximately $300,000. That would leave $100,000 ($400,000 - $300,000) exposed and Eunice would have too much money to qualify for Medicaid. Instead, she can purchase a 2/3 interest in the home ($400,000/$600,000) in exchange for her $400,000. The deed must specifically give Eunice a 2/3 interest in the house, and it must give a right of survivorship to the other owners of the house, so that upon her death her interest passes automatically to Justin and Janice, leaving nothing for the state Medicaid recovery unit to go after (assuming her state does not have an expanded definition of "estate").

NOTE: Not all states permit a right of survivorship among unequal joint owners of real estate.

Joint Interest vs. Life Estate Purchase in Child's Home

The reasons to consider *purchasing* a life estate interest vs. a joint interest in a child's home are similar to those discussed above when comparing the *gift* of a remainder interest and joint interest.

Although the numbers may favor purchasing a life estate interest, one major factor that may or may not make a difference (depending on the parent's health) is that there is no one-year residency requirement for the joint purchase as there is with a life estate purchase. Theoretically, the parent could make the joint interest purchase, move in, and move out to a nursing home the next day, and the interest should still be a valid non-gift transaction. However, the longer the parent actually does reside in the child's home following the purchase, the better it looks to the Medicaid folks and the less trouble the parent will have. After all, the exclusion of the home is based on the parent's "intent to return home," and if the parent only lived there a few days, such claim looks a little flimsy.

Parent's Child Moves into the Home ("Caretaker Child")

See discussion of *Caretaker Child,* Chapter 14.

Parent's Sibling Moves into the Home

See discussion of *Resident Sibling,* Chapter 14

Income Tax Basis of the Home

There are good reasons to make sure your home is included in your taxable estate (i.e., for estate tax purposes). Typically, there is no concern about actually owing estate taxes for anyone thinking about Medicaid eligibility. After all, your estate must exceed $13.99 million (2025 amount) before you will be liable for estate tax (federal), and anyone with that much dough is usually not trying to become Medicaid eligible. However, it is important for *income tax* purposes for your house to be includible in your taxable estate.

There is a federal estate tax rule that says that as long as you retain a right to live in your house for the rest of your life, the house will be includible in your taxable estate for estate tax purposes. As a result, that causes the house to get a new income tax basis equal to the date of death value of the property, which will eliminate any capital gains tax upon a sale of the house immediately following your death. Your right to live in the house does not even have to be in writing; it is enough if there was an implied agreement that you could continue to live there for the rest of your life.

Example:

If you bought your house in 1965 for $50,000 (the *basis*), you gave it away and did not retain the right to live there, and at your death it's worth $350,000, there is a capital gain of $300,000 if the house is sold at that time. Under the current 15% capital gains tax rate, your heirs would be faced with a tax of $45,000! However, if the house were included in your taxable estate, it gets a new income tax basis of $350,000. So if your family sells the house right after your death, they would pay *zero* capital gains tax, saving $45,000.

Reverse Mortgages

Under the federal FHA reverse mortgage rules, a homeowner at least age 62 can borrow against the equity in the house (with a value limit of $1,149,825). There must not be any other debt against the house. The percentage of the equity that can be borrowed depends on the borrower's age and the going interest rate (the older the borrower and the lower the interest rate, the more that can be borrowed). At current interest rates, the amount available is typically between 60% and 70% for borrowers in their 70s and 80s. The loan does not have to be repaid until the homeowner (or remaining spouse) moves, sells the house, or dies.

While a reverse mortgage rarely makes sense for a single person who may soon be applying for Medicaid—because 12 months after a single person moves out of the home the loan must be repaid—it *can* make sense for a couple to apply for one. For example, if one spouse will continue to live in the community while the other spouse is in a nursing home, the Community Spouse may need extra income to pay the bills, modify the home for a wheelchair, purchase a new car, go on trips to visit family members, etc.

Once the loan is approved, the Community Spouse/borrower has three options: withdraw the full amount as a lump sum, leave the amount as a line of credit to be drawn against as needed, or take the loan as an immediate lifetime annuity (or any combination of the foregoing). With the latter, each month the bank or mortgage company sends the Community Spouse a check, hence the name "reverse mortgage." Such payments are not considered "income" that could count against the Community Spouse for Medicaid purposes.

For Medicaid purposes, the house will continue to be an excluded asset, as will the total amount of cash available under the contract. The only time payments will be countable is if they are not spent by the end of the month in which the payment is received. So a lump sum withdrawal will increase the countable assets of the couple and must be carefully planned for: If the loan is taken out *after* the nursing home spouse has qualified for Medicaid, then it should not affect the eligibility of the nursing home spouse, as discussed above.

The total amount of payments made to the Community Spouse under the reverse mortgage contract will eventually have to be repaid, of course, but not until both spouses have left the house, either because of illness, death, or sale of the house. At that time, the house will typically have to be sold to pay off the outstanding loan balance; if the house has decreased in value below the amount due the bank, the bank is out of luck: it cannot go after other estate assets.

Example:

George is age 71, his wife Gracie age 65. Their house is worth $250,000 and has no current debt against it. Regardless of which spouse is in the nursing home, if the Community Spouse takes out a reverse mortgage today, according to one lender consulted, that spouse can receive either (i) a lump sum of $39,189 with a line of credit of $50,000, (ii) a line of credit of $72,189, or (iii) lifetime payments of $474 per month (or any combination of the foregoing). The total borrowed funds do not have to be repaid until the death of the surviving spouse, or, if sooner, when the Community Spouse is forced to move out, e.g., to assisted living or a nursing home. If for any reason they need to sell the house prior to that time, then once again the loan will have to be repaid at that time.

For a helpful reverse mortgage calculator go to:
https://www.reversemortgage.org/about/reverse-mortgage-calculator

Private Reverse Mortgages

A reverse mortgage that meets the FHA rules governing bank-originated reverse mortgages must follow very restrictive rules and can be quite costly, as well. One way to get the benefit of a reverse mortgage but avoid these rules is to implement a private reverse mortgage, i.e., a loan by a family member that is secured by an interest in the home. It would be important for this to be drawn up by an attorney and recorded with the deed, to be sure it is deemed valid by the Medicaid caseworker. This type of arrangement has many benefits:

- If the parent needs additional funds to pay for living expenses, home repairs, or caregivers (including the children) at home or otherwise, this can be a ready source of funds to make their life better. The loan can be in the form of a lump-sum amount or a monthly check.
- Unlike an FHA reverse mortgage, the amount of the loan is not limited to an arbitrary percentage of the value of the house.
- The interest rate payable by the parent back to the family member who makes the loan will often be higher than the low interest rates that banks are paying, enabling the family member making the loan to earn a decent amount of interest on the loan. (The "applicable federal rate" for this type of loan is updated and published by the IRS each month.)
- The interest rate that the parent must pay will normally be lower than what they would otherwise have to pay to the bank.
- You save the high fees that the mortgage company would normally charge to set one of these up.
- Most importantly, unlike an FHA reverse mortgage, the loan need not be paid off within 12 months after the homeowner vacates the house (to move to a nursing home, for example), but can be made due only upon the parents' death or eventual sale of the house.
- Upon the parent's death, the house can be sold and the family member who made the loan repaid out of the proceeds, with accumulated interest.
- Since the loan will be secured by a recorded lien on the house, it will be paid back ahead of the state when the state files its recoupment claim for

estate recovery. That means the family member who made the loan must be paid back in full, with interest, first, and only if there anything left after that will the state be entitled to a portion of the net proceeds from sale of the house, to satisfy its estate recovery claim. NOTE: If the monthly check option is used, then the recorded mortgage document as well as the promissory note itself should include language to account for the additions to the debt over time. This will ensure that the full amount of the loan is secured, so that the debt to the family member can eventually be paid back ahead of the state's claim.

Chapter 12

ANNUITIES

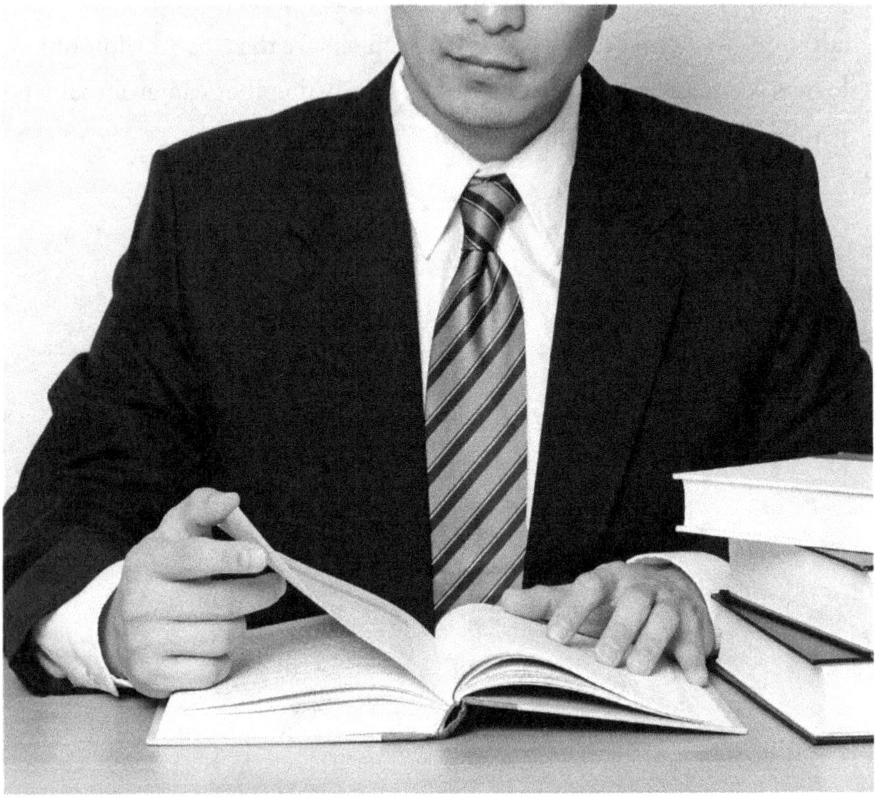

Annuities have become one of the most popular investments in recent years.

In its most basic form, an annuity is an insurance company's contractual agreement to provide payments to the purchaser/ owner at specified intervals over an agreed-upon period of time. The reasons for annuities' popularity are (i) the investment inside the annuity grows on a tax-deferred basis, (ii) the annuity can be set up to continue to pay the owner a fixed amount no matter how long the owner lives and how the stock market performs, and (iii) the investment can have a "guaranteed minimum" return of capital so that the annuity cannot drop below the amount of the initial investment.

In the following discussion, it is important to understand the following terms:

The "**owner**" of an annuity is the person who has the right to change the beneficiary designation of the annuity.

- The "**annuitant**" is the person on whose life expectancy the payments of the annuity are based.
- The "**beneficiary**" is the person or group of persons who receive the annuity payments upon the death of the annuitant. With a Medicaid annuity, beneficiaries only receive such payments *if* there is a "guarantee period" and the annuitant dies before the end of his life expectancy. Otherwise, the payments stop upon the death of the annuitant.
- The "**guarantee period**" is the length of time the annuity payments must be made, whether or not the annuitant survives the entire period. Normally, an annuity would automatically terminate upon the death of the annuitant. However, that could be risky, because you never know how long a person will live. For example, what if the annuitant has a life expectancy of, say, 20 years but dies unexpectedly in year 2? If the annuity payments stop at the death of the annuitant, then most of the money used to purchase that annuity is lost. Instead, had the annuity been purchased with a 20-year guarantee period, then even if the annuitant died in year 2,

payments would continue for the remaining 18 years, to the beneficiaries. Because the company that sells the annuity has greater exposure with an annuity with a guarantee period, the annuity payments will necessarily be lower for the same amount of money invested in the annuity.

- With a **"fixed"** annuity, the owner will receive a check for the same annuity amount every month, regardless of the performance of the stock market. However, with a fixed annuity there is no opportunity to withdraw the principal of the annuity: once the owner purchases the annuity, all they will ever receive back is a series of regular equal payments, for the rest of the annuity term, which could be for a fixed number of years or over the remainder of the owner's life.
- A **"variable"** annuity is invested in the stock market, so that the annuity payments can go up or down, depending on the performance of the underlying investments.
- An **"immediate"** annuity begins to make payments back to the owner immediately following purchase, vs. a **"deferred"** annuity, which is invested and grows and can be tapped by the owner when and as needed.
- The type of annuity that is most common in the non-Medicaid world is the **"deferred variable annuity."** This type of annuity does not have a specific amount that pays out on a regular basis, and it may simply sit there, growing over time, based on market conditions. This is called the
- **"accumulation phase."** At some point, all annuities must make payments, either to the owner, the annuitant, or one or more beneficiaries (after the death of the annuitant); that's called the **"annuitization (or payout) phase."**

Medicaid Planning Annuities

As useful as the foregoing tax and investment benefits may be, in most cases none of these are critical points when considering the use of an annuity for Medicaid planning purposes.

For Medicaid planning, there is a wonderful way to convert countable assets to non-countable: purchase a FIXED, IMMEDIATE ANNUITY. Such an annuity is sometimes referred to as a **"Medicaid Annuity"** or **"Medicaid-friendly Annuity."**

Another type of annuity may start out as a deferred annuity (i.e., payments back to the owner have not yet started) and then convert to an immediate, fixed annuity upon the occurrence of some defined event, such as entering a nursing home. This type may also be called a "Medicaid-friendly Annuity."

Why Annuities Work in Medicaid Planning

The main reason annuities are such a powerful Medicaid planning technique is that once you purchase a "Medicaid annuity," it is no longer a countable asset. Instead, the payments back to the owner are countable solely as payments of income. In effect, you can take $100,000 and buy the right kind of annuity, and suddenly that entire $100,000 has "disappeared" for Medicaid eligibility purposes! However, there are certain rules that must be followed if you want this to work.

General Requirements

In order to avoid having the full purchase price of an annuity be deemed a penalty-causing transfer, a Medicaid annuity *that is not within a retirement plan* must be **fixed, immediate, irrevocable, actuarially sound,** and **nontransferable**.

"Irrevocable" means that once you sign the contract to purchase the annuity, you can neither change its terms nor get your money back.

"Actuarially sound" means that the annuity must not extend past the life expectancy of the annuitant. So either the annuity must pay only for the annuitant's lifetime, or the guarantee period must not be longer than the annuitant's life expectancy.

"Non-transferable" means that you cannot transfer or assign the ownership of the annuity to anyone. You cannot sell it. After all, if you could sell the annuity, then the state Medicaid department could logically demand that you do so, and then apply the proceeds to your nursing home bill. But if the annuity cannot be sold, then it has no value as an asset, other than the stream of income that it pays to you.

By the way, "SPIA" is insurance industry-speak for Single Premium Immediate Annuity, which is the only kind acceptable for Medicaid purposes.

NOTE: Several states have taken the position recently that even though the annuity contract states that it cannot be sold, it still must be valued as a "countable" asset if there are businesses that would sign a contract with the owner of the annuity, exchanging a lump sum payment for an unsecured promise by the owner to pay over each annuity payment as it is received. Although some of the states have lost court cases in this area, it is clearly an evolving area that requires an experienced elder law attorney who is aware of the cases and trends in your own state, to assist you with Medicaid annuity purchases.

Retirement Plan Annuities

An annuity that is wholly owned by a retirement plan is exempt from the above requirements. This will only matter in states where retirement plans are not already exempt resources. This applies to an Individual Retirement Annuity or an annuity established under an employer-sponsored "qualified retirement plan," or an annuity purchased with proceeds from (i) an account or trust described as an IRA, Individual Retirement Trust, or employer-sponsored "qualified retirement plan"; (ii) a simplified employee pension (SEP); or (iii) a Roth IRA. Thus, such an annuity can have a deferred start date and/or unequal payments such as small current payments with a large balloon payment at the end. It still should not exceed the life expectancy of the owner because that will cause a gift under pre-DRA rules, and it still must be irrevocable and non-transferable to avoid being a countable asset under other tests found in the Medicaid rules.

Note that while an annuity within a retirement plan need not be based on the owner's life expectancy in order to qualify as a Medicaid annuity, it must still comply with the minimum distribution rules under the tax code to avoid the 50% tax penalty on smaller-than-required minimum distributions. Accordingly, a retirement plan Medicaid annuity must pay out AT LEAST AS RAPIDLY as that required by the tax code, which is based on the owner's life expectancy. Thus, care must be taken when setting the payout schedule from the annuity so that it meets both the Medicaid AND the IRS rules; otherwise, there would be a 50% tax penalty on the difference between what should have been distributed from the retirement plan (under the minimum distribution rules) and what was actually distributed.

For a single individual these options may not make much of a difference, since the state still must be paid back at the death of the owner, but for a married couple, structuring lower annuity payments up front (or even deferring them) will allow either (i) more income to be shifted from the nursing home spouse to the Community Spouse (see MMMNA rules, above) or (ii) more assets to be protected as part of the CSRA (if the total income of both spouses is less than the MMMNA). Care must be taken to deplete the annuity prior to the death of the Community Spouse, to the extent possible, so as to reduce the amount subject to state repayment of the nursing home spouse's Medicaid costs.

Payback to State

Under the federal Deficit Reduction Act of 2005 (as amended on 12/20/06), effective for all Medicaid annuities issued on or after Feb. 8, 2006, in order to prevent having the purchase of a Medicaid annuity treated as a gift, the state must be named as the successor beneficiary of the annuity payments after the death of the "institutionalized individual," i.e., the person in the nursing home. This is to ensure that the state will be reimbursed out of the remaining annuity payments (if any) for any Medicaid payments it made on behalf of such person.

However, if there is a spouse or a minor or disabled child who is named as the successor beneficiary, then the state must be named as next successor beneficiary after such person(s), and it will have to wait until the death of such person(s) before it can collect on the debt.

Thus, under the above requirement, if the at-home spouse owns a Medicaid annuity and dies survived by the nursing home spouse, the annuity payments must now be made to the state for both the past *and* future Medicaid costs of the nursing home spouse. This means that the contingent beneficiaries (typically the children) must wait until after the death of the surviving spouse to receive any remaining annuity payments.

Single Person Annuity Purchase

Age

Some annuity companies will not issue an annuity based on an annuitant who is over age 85, but others will go as high as 90 or beyond.

Amount

An annuity may be purchased for a single (unmarried) individual in any amount.

Term

If the term of the annuity is based on a life expectancy greater than that of the annuitant, then some portion of the purchase price will be considered a gift, for Medicaid purposes.

Let's take a look at an example

For the rest of this section we are going to follow John, age 65 and unmarried, who because of unfortunate health problems is facing nursing home care for an indefinite period. In order to shelter a portion of his assets, he is considering purchasing a Medicaid annuity. Since he is moving into the nursing home immediately, it's important to him that he does not incur any penalty period.

First, John should look up his life expectancy on the federally published table (see **annuity (Life expectancy) table** at the end of this book). According to this table, a male age 65 has a life expectancy of 16.95 years. Therefore, so long as John purchases an annuity based on his life expectancy, or based on a guaranteed series of equal payments that cannot exceed his life expectancy of 16.95 years (the "guarantee period"), there will be no gift for Medicaid purposes. As a result, the full cost of the annuity will be sheltered and deemed a non-countable asset.

Payments

Each payment to John will be deemed a payment of income in the month received. If any portion of the payment is not spent within the month it is received, such portion will be counted as part of John's assets as of the first day of the following month. If John is in the nursing home at the time the annuity is in effect, then (after deducting some permitted allowances) he must pay the entire amount of each payment to the nursing home.

If John resides in an "income-cap" state, check to see if the annuity payments combined with his other income exceed the income-cap amount. If so, then a Qualified Income Trust will have to be set up to receive either the annuity payments or at least one of his other sources of income, so that he is not disqualified by having too much income during the penalty period (and thereafter, if it continues).

How to Estimate the Monthly Payments

A good estimate of the monthly annuity payments a Medicaid applicant will receive following his or her purchase may be found at this website:

http://www.immediateannuities.com

Here's how to use this website for Medicaid planning purposes:

1. Enter the amount you wish to protect in the box that says "Amount to Invest." Let's assume John wishes to protect $100,000.
2. Select "1 month" under Income to Begin In.

3. Select the age of the Medicaid applicant in the first box on the left.
4. Select the gender and state of residence in the next two boxes to the right.
5. Ignore optional joint-life boxes.
6. Click "Get My Quote." On the next screen, click on the words "Load More Annuity Quotes."
7. Find the Estimated Monthly Income in the table. Look for the guarantee period closest to the Medicaid Table life expectancy. So for John, a male age 65, the life expectancy is 16.9 years (which you got from the Table in the Appendix), so we use the "Life & 15 Years Certain."
8. Since John's life expectancy is between 15 and 20 years, also note the income for "Life & 20 Years Certain."
9. **Summary:** For a male, 65, investing $100,000, the monthly annuity check would be approximately $625 (a little less than halfway between the 15 Years and 20 Years figures.) If the client has no interest in possibly passing on remaining payments after his death to his children (e.g., there will be re-payment to the state, anyway), then he may prefer to go with the single Life option (first one at the top), which pays out slightly more per month.

For a more accurate quote, you will need to contact an agent that sells these types of Medicaid annuities. See the Resources list in the *Appendix* for some suggestions. Alternatively, talk with an experienced elder law attorney in your state who works with an agent who is experienced in selling these types of annuities and who, together with your attorney, can have the annuity set up consistent with the then current Medicaid rules in your state.

Normal Life Expectancy

If John must turn over every annuity payment to the nursing home, and if the payments must stop upon John's death, at first blush it appears that there is no benefit to this type of annuity: at John's death, the annuity payments stop, and no part of the money ever gets to his other family members. However, it may still make sense to purchase an annuity in this case if it will allow John to upgrade to a private room or transfer to a non-Medicaid facility in the future.

Shorter-Than-Normal Life Expectancy

If John's annuity had a guarantee period equal to his life expectancy of 16.9 years, and John dies after, say, five years, the annuity does not stop at his death but must continue for the remainder of the guarantee period, i.e., 11.9 more years. Assume that the monthly payments will be $625 per month.

So if John invested $100,000 in the annuity and turned over every payment he received to the nursing home ($625 per month x 60 months), and he died after five years, his family will receive the balance of the monthly payments for the next 11.9 years: $625 x 12 months x 11.9 years = $89,250.

(NOTE: In most cases the family cannot terminate the annuity and cash it in; they must simply wait and receive each annuity payment according to the same payment schedule that was in effect while John was alive. There are only a few companies that will allow the beneficiaries to cash out; if that is something John wants, then he will have to accept slightly reduced monthly payments in exchange for this option.)

However, if John had qualified for Medicaid coverage, upon his death the annuity payments must go to the state, up to the amount of Medicaid payments it made on John's behalf. So the benefit to his family would have to be reduced accordingly.

If the state must be paid back, does it still make sense to purchase an annuity? It might, *if* certain conditions exist. By qualifying the annuity owner for Medicaid, the payments to the nursing home are reduced. This "stretches out" the benefit of the annuity and reduces the amount of total cost to the family.

Examples:

1. With Estate Recovery Against a Home

If John dies after 5 years

John, age 65, has slightly over $100,000 in countable assets. To qualify for Medicaid, he invests $100,000 in an annuity that will pay him $625 per month for the rest of his life, with a guarantee period of slightly less than his life expectancy of 16.9 years, i.e., 16 years (the guarantee period can never be more than the table life expectancy in order to avoid making a gift). Since his total assets are now under $2,000, he qualifies for Medicaid immediately. His only other income is Social Security of $925 per month. He has a personal needs allowance (PNA) of $35/month, leaving him an $890 patient pay amount (the amount that goes to the nursing home each month). Each month both this patient pay amount and annuity payment must be turned over to the nursing home; Medicaid pays the balance of the bill. If the "Medicaid reimbursement rate" for John's nursing home is $6,500 per month, then each month the state pays the nursing home $6,500 – $890 – $625 = **$4,985**. If John dies after five years, the state will have paid out a total of $299,100 for his care (60 months x $4,985 = $299,100). The state must first be satisfied out of the remaining annuity payments ($625/mo x 12 mos x 11 yrs = $82,500), leaving a balance owed to the state of $216,600. Since John owned a home subject to estate recovery, the state will file a claim for this amount against the home. Assuming the home has a value of at least $216,600, total cost to John and his estate: **$316,600** ($100,000 annuity investment + $216,600 of estate recovery).

Alternatively, if John does not purchase the annuity, in order to reduce his assets below $2,000, he will have to spend down his $100,000 paying the nursing home at the "private pay" rate, of, say $9,000 per month ("Medicaid reimbursement rates" are typically 70% of the private pay rate.) To make the monthly $9,000 payment, he first applies his patient pay amount of $890 and makes up the balance—$8,110—out of his cash savings. Thus his $100,000 will be depleted after a little more than 12 months. At that point he will qualify for Medicaid, and the nursing home cost drops to $6,500 (the Medicaid reimbursement rate). Assuming, again, that John dies after five years, Medicaid will cover him for the next 48 months, until his death, at a cost of $269,280 ([$6,500 – $890] x 48). Again, there is estate recovery against John's home for this amount (assuming it has a value of at least $269,280). Total cost to John and his estate: **$369,280** ($100,000 assets + $269,280 of estate recovery).

As you can see, by purchasing the annuity, even though no part of that annuity money will ever be paid to other family members, ***John's family***

saves up to $52,680 ($369,280 - $316,600) because the estate recovery bill has been reduced.

If John lives to his full life expectancy of 18 years

If John purchases the annuity, he qualifies for Medicaid immediately and must pay the nursing home at the Medicaid reimbursement rate ($6,500/month). Upon his death 16.9 years later, the amount owed to the state will be $4,985/mo x 12 mos x 16.9 yrs = $1,010,958. Had he not purchased the annuity, he would have first used up his $100,000 in one year and then Medicaid would have paid the full amount for the next 15.9 years ([$6,500 – $890]/mo x 12 mos x 15.9 yrs = $1,070,388).

Since the annuity was depleted long before his death, the state can only seek recovery against his estate, which consists solely of his house. So, depending on the value of his house at the time of his death, the annuity purchase may or may not ultimately save his family any money: if his house is worth no more than the amount owed the state after the annuity purchase ($1,010,958 in our example), his family breaks even (that is, they didn't save any money by John buying the annuity, but they didn't lose any money, either). But if his house is worth more than the amount owed the state at his death, then his family will come out ahead (in our example, they can save up to that same amount as above, $52,680). Thus, there's not much downside risk to purchasing the annuity, and there's a lot of upside potential!

NOTE: The older John is at the time he purchases the annuity and the more valuable his house, the more likely it is that there will be money left for his family following a full repayment of the state at his death, meaning that his family will have benefited from the annuity option. In all cases, any savings may be limited by the value of the house in John's estate. But as long as the house is worth at least as much as the amount owed the state in the annuity purchase option, there will be savings for the family (up to the amounts indicated above).

2. With No Estate Recovery Against a Home

If John died after five years and had no assets in his name at the time of his death, then it made no difference whether he had purchased the annuity or not: either he spent his $100,000 and then qualified for Medicaid or he purchased the annuity, qualified for Medicaid sooner, but then lived long enough to run up a bill owed to the state at least equal to the value of the remaining annuity payments. In either case, his family receives nothing at his death.

But purchasing the annuity may still make sense, if John has a much shorter-than-normal life expectancy. For example, if he died after only one year, then the reduction in the nursing home costs by paying the Medicaid reimbursement rate—as opposed to the private pay rate—would indeed have saved the family money, even assuming full repayment to the state. Here's how the numbers would work out:

Without the annuity: Each month John pays the nursing home $9,000 ($8,110 of his cash + $890 [Social Security – PNA]). After 12 months he has paid them $108,000.

With the annuity: Each month John pays the nursing home $890 + $625 (from the annuity) and Medicaid pays the difference between that and the $6,500 Medicaid rate, i.e., $6,500 – 890 – 625 = $4,985. If he dies after one year, a portion of his remaining annuity payments will be used to pay back the state for its 12 months of payments (12 mos x $4,985/mo = $59,820), with the balance passing to his family. He paid the nursing home directly 12 x (890 + 625) = $18,180. So between what he paid directly and what the state must be paid back following his death, the total cost is $78,000 ($59,820 + $18,180).

So, in effect, **his family saved $30,000** ($108,000 - $78,000).

Another way of looking at it is that by purchasing the annuity John saved his family $2,500 per month, since by purchasing the annuity John qualified for Medicaid immediately and thus was charged the lower Medicaid reimbursement rate of $6,500 vs. the private pay rate of $9,000. Result: 12 mos x $2,500/mo = **$30,000 saved**.

To summarize, if a single individual has no other assets other than the Medicaid annuity, **the breakeven point is as follows:** once the amount owed to the state equals or exceeds the value of the remaining annuity payments, there is no longer any benefit to having purchased the annuity. In other words, as long as the total of the remaining annuity payments exceeds the balance owed the state upon the death of the annuitant, the family will come out ahead. But again, there is no downside to having purchased the annuity. Since one never is sure how long a person will live, if there is any reasonable possibility that the annuity will save money for the family, it is worth purchasing.

BOTTOM LINE FOR UNMARRIED INDIVIDUALS: The purchase of a Medicaid annuity for a single individual should definitely be considered as an option when the individual owns a home that might be subject to estate recovery. Such purchase would be particularly attractive if the potential Medicaid applicant has a shorter-than-normal life expectancy. Even if the individual does not own a home, the annuity purchase can be beneficial if the individual has a much shorter-than-normal life expectancy. Finally, often a combination of a gift and an annuity will make sense where purchase of an annuity alone will not (see Half-a-Loaf planning discussion, below).

Half-a-Loaf vs. Annuity Only: Whether to use a combination of a gift with a smaller annuity purchase (the "half-a-loaf" plan) or simply a larger annuity purchase without making a gift depends on the facts of each case and the difference between the actual life expectancy of the Medicaid applicant and what the tables say his or her life expectancy should be. There simply is no way to know which plan is better without running the numbers for each scenario and weighing the probabilities. Because of the complexity (as you can see, above!), it is helpful to hire an experienced elder law attorney with a specialty in Medicaid planning when working through these options.

Married Couple Annuity Purchase

With a married couple you can either base the annuity period on the age of the spouse in the nursing home or on that of the Community Spouse. However, under the federal DRA law enacted in 2006, as amended in December 2006 by the Tax Relief and Health Care Act of 2006, the state must be named as a beneficiary of the annuity, so that it can be reimbursed for any Medicaid benefits it paid on behalf of the "institutionalized individual."

So if the nursing home spouse purchases an annuity and dies, the full amount of Medicaid payments the state made on that spouse's behalf must be paid back out of the remaining annuity payments, to the extent of their value (although if there is a surviving spouse or a minor or disabled child named as successor beneficiary, the state will have to wait until the death of such person(s) to collect on this debt. This cannot necessarily be avoided by having the Community Spouse purchase the annuity and receive the annuity payments, since the amount of Medicaid payments made on behalf of the nursing home spouse must *still* be paid back—out of the annuity—upon the death of the Community Spouse.

However, if the annuity payments have stopped during the lifetime of the Community Spouse, then there will be no remainder available at the death of the Community Spouse from which to repay the state.

Thus, it will normally make the most sense to purchase as short an annuity as possible, if the Community Spouse is going to be the recipient of the annuity payments.

Note that if the Community Spouse is the owner of the annuity and is receiving monthly payments, if the Community Spouse him- or herself winds up in the nursing home at some point in the future, the state rules may require that the beneficiary designation name the state so it can be reimbursed for any Medicaid benefits it paid on behalf of the "institutionalized individual," which is now the Community Spouse. If the state was only named the beneficiary as to payments it made on behalf of the *nursing home spouse* and not the Community Spouse, it may require that the beneficiary designation be changed. The literal language of the new federal amendment seems to indicate that the state need only be repaid for the costs of the person who is the "institutionalized individual" *at the time of the annuity purchase.* By definition, the Community Spouse is never an "institutionalized individual" at the time of the annuity purchase. However, you will need to check your own state's regulations (i.e., talk with an elder law attorney) before you actually purchase a Medicaid annuity for a married person.

Another reason to have the annuity payments made to the Community Spouse is so that the payments are not "wasted" by having them paid to the nursing home, as they must be with an unmarried person's annuity. Since all of the annuity payments are made to the Community Spouse, and the income of the Community Spouse never has to be transferred to the nursing home spouse, 100% of the annuity money can essentially be retained by the family unit, while permitting the nursing home spouse immediately to qualify for Medicaid.

Possible Gift if MMMNA Exceeded

The only consideration is that the annuity period may not exceed the life expectancy of the annuitant spouse (such as the Community Spouse) without causing a gift. This is the same rule as applies to an annuity purchased for a single individual, discussed above.

In some states, if the annuity payment to the Community Spouse causes the income of that spouse to exceed the MMMNA, then the portion of the annuity that causes such excess will be considered a gift (to the named beneficiaries of the annuity, which is typically the children). This would apply only to the extent that the gifted amount causes the CSRA to exceed the maximum (currently $154,140), but typically a Medicaid annuity would not be purchased unless there *were* excess assets: after all, the main purpose of buying the annuity was to convert those excess countable assets into a non-countable annuity.

In such a state, the lower the income of both spouses, the greater the amount of the annuity that can be purchased without creating a gift that causes a penalty period. Unfortunately, smaller monthly payments means a longer annuity period, which is the opposite of what you normally would want: as discussed above, the shorter the annuity payout period, the less chance the state will ever get paid back for the Medicaid payments it made on behalf of the nursing home spouse. Remember, it's only the annuity payments continuing after the Community Spouse's death that the state can tap into for repayment.

Effect on Community Spouse's Income

The Community Spouse is entitled to a minimum amount of income per month, under federal law. Until July 1, 2025, this amount—known as the Minimum Monthly Maintenance Needs Allowance ("MMMNA")—is $2,555 (slightly higher in AK and HI). If the Community Spouse's income (from Social Security, pensions, etc.) is less than this amount, then the Institutionalized Spouse is entitled to shift the amount necessary to bring the Community Spouse up to this amount, from the income of the nursing home spouse. (See detailed discussion of these rules in Chapter 6)

So *if the Community Spouse's income is less than the MMMNA*, and that income is suddenly increased following the purchase of a Medicaid annuity, then that can reduce or eliminate the ability to shift income from the nursing home spouse to the Community Spouse. As a result, more of the couple's joint income will be "wasted" in paying for nursing home care that Medicaid otherwise would have paid for. This result must be considered and brought into any calculation of the benefits of having the Community Spouse purchase a Medicaid annuity.

Notwithstanding the above, an annuity may still be worth purchasing because it can continue after the death of the nursing home spouse. If the Community Spouse were relying on the income of the nursing home spouse as a supplement, that income will typically end upon the death of the nursing home spouse. The income from the annuity, however, will almost always continue for the lifetime of the Community Spouse. So it is a more reliable, long-term benefit, all other things being equal.

Example:

Martha lives in the community while her husband, Daniel, is in the nursing home. They own a home and have countable assets of $200,000. Martha's only income is $1,000 per month from Social Security; each month Daniel receives $600 from a pension that terminates at his death and Social Security of $900. Under the MMMNA rules discussed above, once Daniel is covered by Medicaid Martha would be entitled to at least $2,555 of income per month. Since her income is less than that, she would be entitled to shift some of her husband's income over to her to bring her income up to $2,555. Thus, she would be entitled to all $1,500 of Daniel's income and Medicaid would pick up the balance of his nursing home bill.

However, this couple won't qualify for Medicaid because they have approximately $100,000 of excess assets. So Martha decides to convert the extra $100,000 to a Medicaid annuity. At age 71 she can purchase an annuity that does not exceed her table life expectancy of 15 years (if it is for longer than that, part of the purchase price will be deemed a gift to her children). After checking with a few annuity companies, she found out that if she wants to receive payments for the remainder of her life with a 15-year minimum payout, the most she can receive each month on a $100,000 annuity investment would be $683.

Since her income from Social Security is $1,000, the annuity payments will increase her income to $1,683 per month. As a result, this will reduce the amount she would otherwise be entitled to shift from Daniel's income to herself by $683 per month. Under these new facts she would be entitled to $872 of Danielle's income and the remaining $628 (minus the $160 Personal Needs Allowance) would be paid to the nursing home. In a way, the amount of Daniel's income she *could* have shifted to herself is "wasted," in that now it must be paid to the nursing home, where all it will accomplish is a reduction of what Medicaid has to pay. However, this plan still makes sense, because it permits Daniel to qualify for Medicaid immediately. In addition, upon Daniel's death, his pension and Social Security will terminate, and if their extra $100,000 of assets had been spent on his nursing home care instead of used to purchase the annuity, Martha's income would then drop back to $1,000 and not remain at $1,683 for the rest of her life.

Effect on Community Spouse's Assets (CSRA)

If the total income of *both* spouses is less than the MMMNA, having income from a Medicaid annuity paid to the Community Spouse could prevent the ability to protect additional assets under the theory that such assets would be needed to generate additional income (by a Fair Hearing to increase the CSRA, as discussed in Chapter 7). Indeed, if the couple's income is low enough—or if the MMMNA can be increased enough—it may be possible for the Community Spouse to protect sufficient additional assets this way without needing to purchase an annuity at all. If it is possible to protect additional assets by increasing the CSRA, that is preferable to purchasing a Medicaid annuity, since, among other things, there would be no payback requirement to the state following the death of the surviving spouse.

Deciding on the Length of the Annuity Term

There are competing goals in deciding the length of the annuity term. To minimize the income of the Community Spouse, you want the annuity to be for as long a period of time as possible without causing it to be a gift, i.e., up to the full "table" life expectancy of the Community Spouse. That's because the longer the term, the lower each monthly payment to the Community Spouse. And the lower the Community Spouse's income, the more income that can be shifted from the nursing home spouse. Indeed, if after each annuity payment the total income of both spouses is still below the MMMNA, additional assets can be sheltered as part of the CSRA (thereby reducing the amount of the annuity needed). However, the longer the annuity term the greater the possibility that the Community Spouse will die before receiving all of the annuity payments. As discussed above, that could expose those payments to a repayment claim of the state.

In order to figure out what to do, first look at the income of the Community Spouse (Social Security plus pensions, etc.). If it's *above* the MMMNA (and remember, that can be adjusted above the minimum, in certain cases), then you might as well get as short an annuity as you can, since in that situation there's no way to shift additional income or assets to the Community Spouse. If the

Community Spouse's income is *below* the MMMNA, then you have to look at the amount of income or assets that can be shifted and balance that against the life expectancy of the Community Spouse: the longer the Community Spouse is expected to live (relative to his or her "table" life expectancy), the more sense it makes to get a longer-term annuity. That may permit shifting income (and possibly sheltering additional assets, too) without too much risk that the Community Spouse will die before receiving most or all of the annuity payments. (If the payment period is for the longer of a guaranteed term of years *or* the life of the Community Spouse, then it only matters if the Community Spouse dies before the end of the guarantee period; after that, whether or not the Community Spouse has actually lived to his or her full life expectancy is irrelevant, because the payments will end at the Community Spouse's death, leaving nothing for repayment to the state.)

Calculating the Gift

If an annuity is purchased with a guarantee period longer than the life expectancy of the annuitant, then the amount of money attributable to the excess payments is deemed a gift to the named beneficiaries. So if your life expectancy is 15 years, and you purchase a Medicaid annuity payable to you with a guarantee period of 20 years, then you have made a gift equal to the difference between the cost of an annuity with a 15-year guarantee period and total cost of the purchased annuity. As a general rule, it makes more sense simply to make a current outright gift of that excess amount rather than purchase a longer annuity, because the annuity purchase incurs a significant commission cost, ties up the money inside the annuity, and subjects an additional amount to possible state payback.

Annuity Purchase by the Community Spouse

One method of reducing a couple's total assets by a large amount is to have the Community Spouse (i.e., the healthy spouse) purchase a large annuity prior to the other spouse needing to apply for Medicaid. If a portion of such purchase will be deemed a gift (see next paragraph), then the purchase should be completed at least five years prior to applying for Medicaid, so that once the five-year lookback period has passed, the gift will be ignored. And, since the annuity payments to the Community Spouse are not attributable to the nursing home spouse, the Community Spouse will essentially get the benefit of the entire amount of money used to purchase the annuity. In other words, even though it may be deemed a gift for Medicaid eligibility purposes, in reality, the purchasing spouse is retaining all the payments of income (i.e., the annuity payments) back to him- or herself.

It should be made clear that there are only two situations when such a purchase will result in a gift: (i) in those states where an annuity payment causes the Community Spouse's income to exceed the MMMNA and (ii) if the annuity has a guarantee period that exceeds the Community Spouse's life expectancy (see prior section, *"Calculating the Gift"*). In either of such cases, the purchase of the annuity will result in some portion of the purchase price being deemed a gift, and therefore the five-year lookback period must be considered.

In all other cases, the Community Spouse can use the full amount of excess assets (i.e., the full "spenddown" amount) to purchase a Medicaid annuity payable to the Community Spouse, and not have to worry about the lookback period since such purchase will *not* be deemed a gift. Thus, it can be used at any time, right up until a Medicaid application is filed, and thus must be considered a valuable "crisis" planning technique.

How Large Can the Annuity Be?

Although there is no theoretical limit on the amount of assets that can be sheltered this way, there is a practical limit. For example, if a couple has $500,000 of excess resources and the healthy spouse purchases a Medicaid annuity payable to himself five years in advance of his wife applying for Medicaid, it's true that, by the time of the Medicaid application, the $500,000 annuity will be ignored, since it was purchased outside of the five-year lookback period. However, the monthly annuity payment may be so large that the Community Spouse does not spend it all each month, so that by the time the wife applies for Medicaid, some of those payments have accumulated, causing the couple to have excess resources, again. As a result, the wife will not be eligible for Medicaid until those excess resources are spent down or otherwise disposed of. (Of course, it may be possible for the Community Spouse to buy another Medicaid annuity at that time, in the amount of the excess accumulated assets!)

Long-Term Care Insurance Option

What if the couple is concerned that the less-healthy spouse may need to enter a nursing home prior to the expiration of the five-year period, following the annuity purchase? In that case, the couple should consider immediately purchasing long-term care insurance for the less-healthy spouse, if at all possible. It is a good way to hedge one's bets, particularly when health is still good currently, but you are doing some long-term planning. If the health of the ill spouse precludes purchasing a long-term care insurance policy, then the couple should be sure to retain sufficient assets in addition to the CSRA to cover the anticipated cost of the nursing home, for the period prior to the expiration of the five-year lookback period. You don't want to retain *too* many assets, however, in case it turns out that the ill spouse didn't need nursing home care as soon as you thought, leaving you with excess assets at the end of the lookback period. As you can see, this involves guessing how long it may be before the less healthy spouse may need to move to a nursing home, so you need to consider all the different possible scenarios when deciding how much to set aside.

Planning for the Community Spouse Entering a Nursing Home

As explained above, when planning for the possible need for nursing home care of the Community Spouse at some point after the annuity purchase, there may or may not be a five-year lookback period to worry about. More critical will be the amount of each monthly annuity payment to the Community Spouse, since such payments, when added to the other income of the Community Spouse (e.g., Social Security and pension payments), may exceed the state's maximum income requirements to qualify for Medicaid.

Thus, a smaller annuity payment may be more prudent, when considering a possible future Medicaid application for the Community Spouse, in order to keep the Community Spouse's total income under the state's maximum allowable amount.

Recent Developments

Although specifically permitted under federal law, the so-called "Medicaid annuity" discussed above allows so much money to be converted from countable to non-countable that a number of states have passed laws restricting their use. One type of restriction has already been discussed, that of limiting the amount of the annuity for a Community Spouse to that necessary to increase the Community Spouse's income to the MMMNA, by treating any excess as a gift or requiring it to be paid to the nursing home. Indeed, a number of federal appeals courts have recently held that state regulations capping the amount of funds an applicant for Medicaid benefits may use to purchase a Medicaid annuity for the benefit of the community spouse at the CSRA limit "is invalid because it is inconsistent with federal law." If you are in a state with such a regulation, you should consider asking your attorney if he or she is willing to challenge the state regulation; there seem to be sufficient cases out there, now, in support of such a change. If you have enough assets to protect, this could be well worth pursuing in court.

In a recent Connecticut case the court refused to characterize the income stream from a Medicaid annuity as an asset. In this case, the annuity payments were irrevocable and non-assignable and were paid to the at-home spouse so that the nursing home spouse could qualify for Medicaid. The state Medicaid department attempted to count the annuity payment stream as an asset that could be sold, which would have disqualified the spouse in the nursing home from qualifying for Medicaid. However, both the lower court and the Appeals Court (as well as the brief filed by U.S. Department of Health and Human Services) refused to go along with that interpretation, and they held that it's clear in the law that such payments are income and not assets for Medicaid eligibility purposes.

Other states have attempted to restrict the use of Medicaid annuities by requiring that even non-transferable annuities must be valued as if they could be sold on the open market. Once again, it is absolutely necessary to have a local elder law attorney discuss this with you, so that you will know whether or not these techniques are available in your state.

IRAs and Converting to an Annuity

In most states, when a single individual applies for Medicaid, an IRA or other tax-deferred retirement plan owned by the individual will have to be liquidated, unless it can be annuitized (see below). For married couples, if the nursing home spouse has an IRA, it is possible in some states to convert the IRA into a "Medicaid annuity" and pay the annuity directly to the Community Spouse. By naming the Community Spouse as the payee of the annuity, the income is deemed owned by the Community Spouse. Under the Medicaid annuity rules the IRA is no longer countable as an asset owned by the nursing home spouse.

It is usually possible to convert an IRA into an annuity without having to withdraw the entire amount of the IRA. You will need to discuss this with your financial advisor or IRA administrator, who probably will not be familiar with Medicaid annuity planning. If so, you should show them the discussion in this book and make sure they also check with an experienced elder law attorney. The main advantage of this conversion is that the IRA will be counted as an income stream to the payee (either the nursing home resident—if unmarried—or the Community Spouse, if any) and the IRA itself will no longer be counted as a disqualifying asset.

Although the annuity need not be paid to the IRA owner, it nonetheless must be based on the owner's life expectancy. To decide if the IRA should be annuitized or simply withdrawn requires an analysis of the Medicaid annuity rules in the context of the Medicaid applicant's entire financial and health situation. See the first part of this chapter for further discussion of annuity planning.

If the IRA is owned by the Community Spouse, it should be retained if at all possible, due to its tax advantages. However, if retaining it still causes the couple's assets to be too high, then some part or all of it may have to be liquidated to allow for gifting or other techniques discussed in this book, unless—once again—it can be annuitized.

If the IRA is so large that part of it will be taxed in a higher bracket than the rest of the IRA owner's income, then try to spread the withdrawals out over more than one calendar year, so as to reduce the overall tax bill. If you need to reduce the Medicaid applicant's or spouse's assets in as short a time period as possible, then deferring the total withdrawal of the IRA may not make sense: you will probably wind up paying more to the nursing home for the extra months the Medicaid applicant is disqualified from Medicaid than you'll save in income taxes from the deferral into a second calendar year. (An exception is the Roth IRA: since this was taxed when the IRA converted to the Roth IRA, there is no tax upon withdrawal.)

Private Annuities

A "private annuity" is simply an annuity arrangement between family members, as opposed to a commercial annuity involving an insurance company. The big advantage with a private annuity is that if the family member on whose life the annuity payments are based dies early, it means that the family will keep all the payments that did not have to be made. With a commercial annuity, if the person receiving the annuity payments dies earlier than expected, then—depending on the type of annuity you purchased—the payments stop and the insurance company profits at the family's expense.

Since not all states allow the use of a private annuity, be sure to check before you set one of these up among family members.

Balloon Payment

With an unmarried Medicaid recipient, every payment of the annuity must go either to the nursing home or to allowable medical expenses, reducing what Medicaid would otherwise have paid. So for a Medicaid recipient with no other assets, it really does not benefit the family at all unless the recipient dies before his or her "table" life expectancy, i.e., the number of years the Medicaid recipient is "expected" to live based on the federally mandated life expectancy tables used for these purposes. As a result, the smaller the monthly payments, the more will be available to go to family members upon the nursing home resident's death.

One way to achieve this is to reduce the monthly payments to a very low amount, with the difference being added to a single large final payment just before the expiration of the nursing home resident's life expectancy. Because the payment amount "balloons" in size for that final payment, this is known as a "balloon payment" annuity. However, the Deficit Reduction Act passed in 2006 disqualifies any annuity contract (other than a retirement plan annuity or an annuity purchased outside the five-year lookback period—see discussions above) that includes a "balloon" payment option, so this technique is only useful in rare circumstances.

Chapter 13

PROMISSORY NOTES

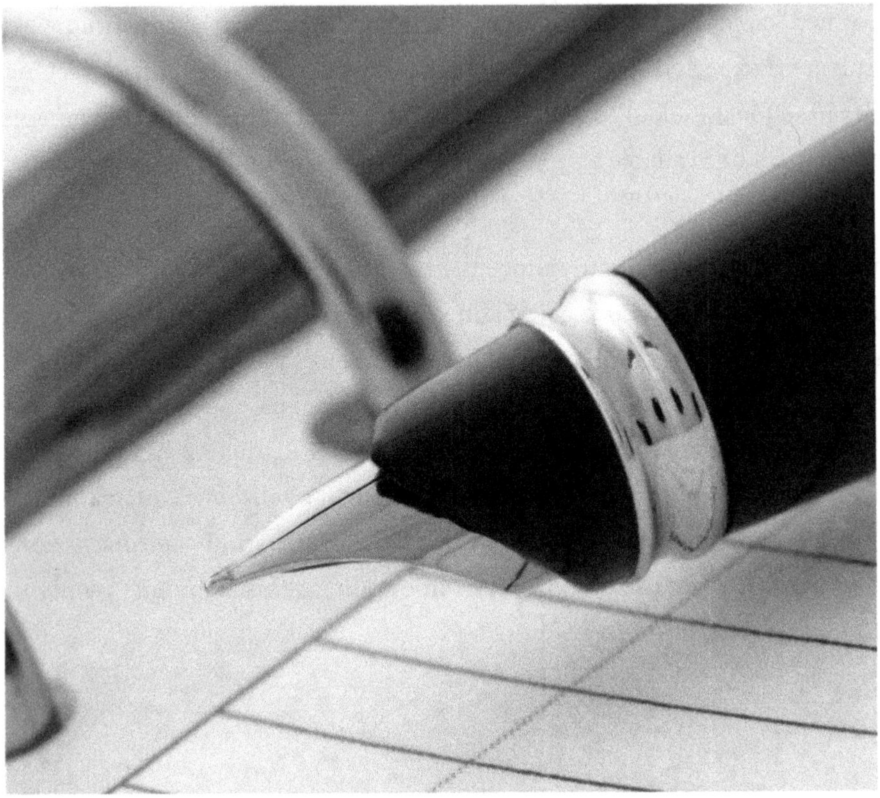

A "promissory note" or "note" is simply an IOU. For Medicaid planning purposes, a properly structured promissory note is ignored, meaning that you can convert an asset that was available to an asset that is not available for Medicaid purposes by lending it to someone else!

The promissory note must meet the following requirements for this to work:

1. It cannot require payments over a period of time longer than the life expectancy of the lender;
2. All payments must be equal in amount; and
3. The note cannot be cancelable upon the lender's death.

In order to avoid having the loan from the person in the nursing home counted as a gift of the entire amount loaned, there must be a promissory note documenting the loan. It should set out the names of the lender and the borrower, the amount of the loan, the term of the loan (i.e., how long until the loan must be completely repaid), the amount of each payment back to the lender, the amount of interest charged (if any), etc.

To avoid challenge by the state that the note is a sham and therefore will be deemed a gift, the note must be bona fide, which means that the loan must be (1) enforceable under state law, (2) in effect at the time the cash proceeds were provided, (3) include an acknowledgment of an obligation to repay, (4) a plan for repayment, (5) the repayment plan must be feasible, and (6) made in good faith (and not merely to qualify for Medicaid). In a 2011 case, the court held that the note was not bona fide, because the son (the borrower) was not credit worthy and there was no security or collateral for the loan. In other words, it was not feasible that it would be repaid. Thus, the loan was treated as a disqualifying transfer (gift) from parent to child.

Length of Payment Term

If the lender is to be the family member in the nursing home, then the smaller each payment back to the lender, the better. After all, the payment will simply be applied to the nursing home bill and only serve to reduce what Medicaid pays the nursing home. In other words, it won't benefit the family member in the nursing home.

You might be tempted to stretch out the payments over, say, a 40-year period, even if the family member in the nursing home is 85. After all, the greater the number of payments, the smaller each payment will be. However, to avoid making a gift that will cause the family member to be disqualified from receiving Medicaid for a period of time, the term of the loan cannot exceed the life expectancy of the lender at the time the loan is made. To find the correct life expectancy, you use the same table used for annuity purchases (see **annuity (Life expectancy) table** in the appendix).

Example:

Lulu resides in a nursing home and has $51,000 in her bank account and no other assets. To qualify for Medicaid, Lulu decides to lend $50,000 to her son, so she can then immediately apply for Medicaid. Because Lulu is age 70, you would look at the Annuity (Life Expectancy) Tables for Female Life Expectancy, age 70. The table indicates that her life expectancy is 16 years. This means that the loan must be repaid within this time period. Converting this to months, it means that the loan cannot exceed a total of 191 months. If you wind up with a fraction of a month, to be conservative always round down to the nearest whole month.

Equal Payments

Once you know how long the loan will last (i.e., its "term"), it's a simple matter to determine the amount of each monthly payment: divide the amount of the loan by the number of months of the term.

Example:

Lulu's life expectancy is 192 months, so divide the amount of the loan—$50,000—by 192, to get $260.42. This figure represents the amount that the lender must pay to Lulu each month, for the term of the loan: 192 months. (This assumes no interest is charged.)

Other Important Clauses of the Note

- **Non-cancelable:** The note must prohibit cancellation upon the death of the lender.
- **Name a beneficiary:** If the laws of your state permit it, and recovery is only permitted against the probate estate, then the note itself should name a successor to whom the payments will be made upon the death of the lender. This will avoid having the note payments flow through the probate estate of the lender. As a result, the state's right of recovery will be defeated.
- If your state does not permit this, the remaining payments must be made to the estate of the lender, where they will be subject to a recovery claim by the state (see Chapter 16). If your state has adopted the expanded definition of "estate", then this will not matter, since the unpaid balance of the note will be subject to estate recovery in either case.
- **Non-assignable:** The note must state that it cannot be pledged, canceled, or assigned by the lender. It should also state that if it *is* sold, transferred, or assigned, such sale, transfer, or assignment will be void and will have no value. If the note cannot be sold, transferred or pledged as collateral for a loan, then its only value is as a stream of income, *not* as an asset, and the state cannot claim otherwise.

Interest Rate Charged

There is no requirement that a certain amount of interest be charged for the loan. As a general rule, it is probably best not to charge *any* interest. That reduces the amount of each payment back to the lender (the parent) and simplifies the calculations, too.

However, if less interest is charged than what the federal government says is the going rate for a loan of the type you've signed then there are income tax consequences. The difference between the interest you charged—if any—and the amount the government says is the going rate at the time of your loan, is known as "foregone" interest, and it is treated as taxable income to the lender as if the lender actually received the money. There is an exception for loans that do not exceed $10,000, so long as the borrowed funds are not directly used to buy income-producing assets (such as stocks or bonds). Also, for loans between two people that do not exceed $100,000 in the aggregate, the amount of imputed interest cannot exceed the borrower's net investment income for the year. Net investment income is basically interest, dividends, and short-term capital gains, less any investment expense, but if the net investment income of the borrower for any year does not exceed $1,000, then the net investment income of the borrower for the year is treated as zero.

In addition, the foregone interest for each year is treated as a *taxable gift* from the lender to the borrower. This will almost always be under the $18,000 annual exclusion for people attempting to qualify for Medicaid. Also, no actual out-of-pocket federal gift tax will have to be paid by the lender unless the total amount of taxable lifetime gifts made by the lender exceeds $13.99 million (2025 amount)!

Thus, if no interest is being paid to the lender, there are two results: (i) there is an "imputed" interest payment to the lender from the borrower, and (ii) there is a deemed *gift* of the imputed interest from the lender *to* the borrower, as if made on the last day of each calendar year. Luckily, there are monetary loan limits under which the imputed interest is treated as zero. These can be very complex to calculate.

Bottom line: It's best to consult an accountant to help you figure out the imputed income, to avoid getting in trouble with the IRS!

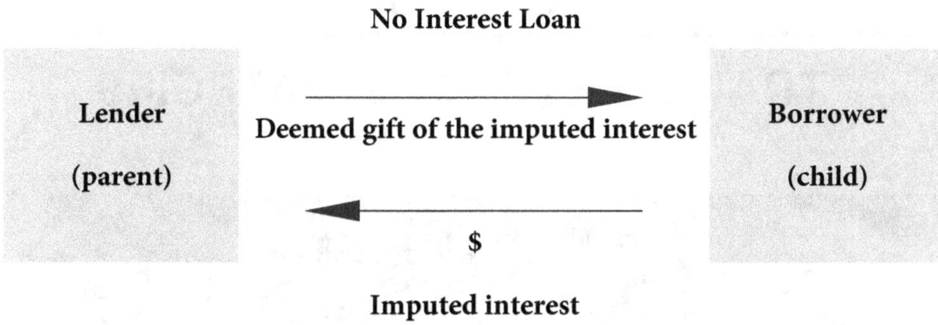

Recent Developments

Some states have begun to institute regulations that characterize promissory notes as countable resources, even if they meet the requirements listed above. Although this seems directly to contradict the federal statute, it points out once again the hazards of trying to do these techniques on your own, without the advice of an experienced and up-to-date elder law attorney.

If it turns out that your state has not issued regulations on the treatment of promissory notes for Medicaid eligibility purposes, you may decide to follow the federal rules and hope for the best. However, if the Medicaid administrators in your state later decide that what you did doesn't work as you planned, you may wind up as a "test case," causing you to incur legal expenses as you attempt to defend your interpretation of the rules, and possibly setting you back to square one if you lose! Thus, caution is in order unless there is already a clear path of regulations addressing this issue in your state.

Chapter 14

TRANSFER (GIFT) STRATEGIES

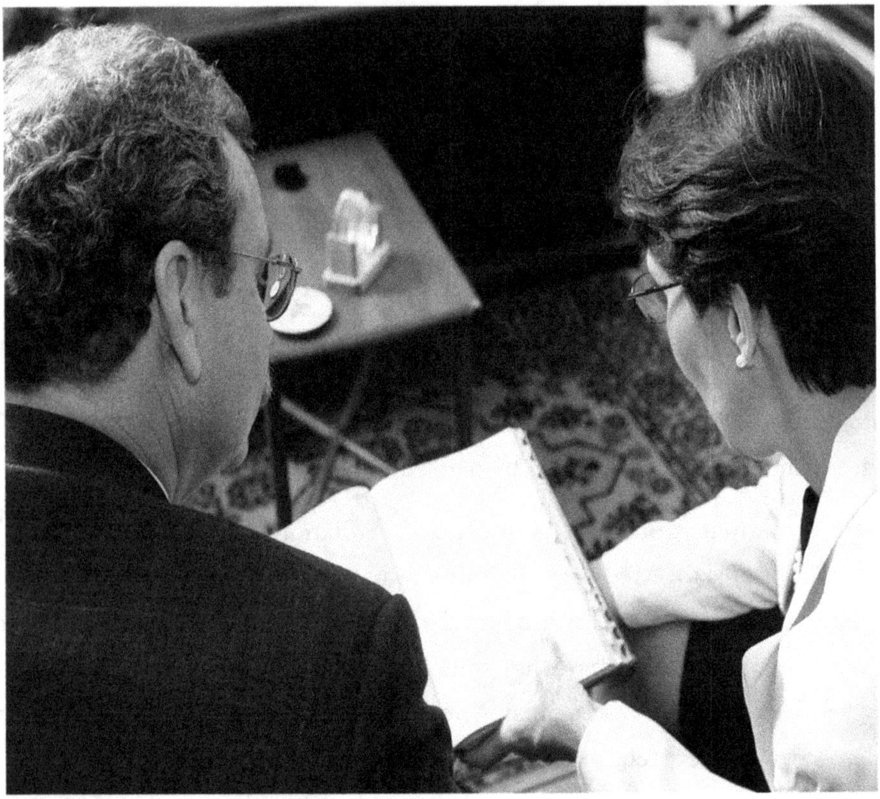

The "Half-a-Loaf" Method

A very popular method of spending down excess resources was known as the "half-a-loaf" method. Although this must now be modified due to the changes implemented by the DRA, when this was first conceived a number of years ago, it worked like this: you give away approximately half of your countable assets, which results in a penalty period. However, you can now use the other half to pay for your living expenses or nursing home costs during this period. At the end of the penalty period, you should just run out of money, so that now you can apply for and qualify for Medicaid coverage.

Example:

Roland is about to enter a nursing home. He has $102,000 in the bank and his only income is Social Security of $1,000 per month. The nursing home costs $6,000 per month, meaning that it's reducing his bank account by $5,000 per month ($6,000 total cost – $1,000 income). At the rate of $5,000 a month, if Roland does no planning, he will have spent $100,000 in 20 months, leaving him with only $2,000. At that point, he will be able to qualify for Medicaid coverage of his nursing home expenses.

But Roland will have spent all his money. Instead, Roland gives away all of his money to his children ($100,000), except for the $2,000 exclusion amount. Assuming the state penalty divisor is $5,000, this will result in a penalty period of 20 months. In other words, he cannot qualify for Medicaid coverage for 20 months after the date he made this gift. Who will pay the nursing home during this time? Unfortunately, his children, recipients of the gift, will have to use the very money Roland just gave them, to pay the nursing home for the penalty period. At the end of the 20 months, Roland will be past the penalty period, and since he will only have $2,000, he will then qualify for Medicaid. But it took the full $100,000 of his money, leaving his children with nothing.

As you can see, **there is no benefit to Roland giving away all his money to his children,** because they'll just have to turn around and use that money to pay for his nursing home care during the resulting penalty period.

The half-a-loaf method is a vast improvement, saving him approximately half of his money. Here's how it works:

Roland gives his children not $100,000, but half that amount, or $50,000. That results in a 10-month penalty period ($50,000 ÷ $5,000 = 10). Roland still has $52,000 left, so he simply pays the nursing home himself, for the 10-month period. At the end of the 10 months, the penalty period expires, and Roland is down to just $2,000. At that point, he can immediately apply for Medicaid coverage and based on his assets and income, he should qualify. Result? He only had to wait 10 months, not 20, and his children have the $50,000 that Roland gave them.

Amount saved: $50,000.

Unfortunately, the numbers almost never work out as cleanly as the above. Accordingly, there is a formula you can use to calculate the proper amount to give away. In the following, "income" includes only regularly occurring income such as Social Security, pension, Railroad Retirement, etc. It does not include interest and dividends from the bank accounts or other investments of the person applying for Medicaid.

The Half-a-Loaf Formula

[Countable assets ÷ (A + B) = # of months penalty] x B = amount to transfer

Explanation of Formula:
Countable assets ÷ (net monthly expenses + state penalty divisor) = number of months penalty. Multiply that number by the state penalty divisor = amount to transfer.

Start with the **total amount of countable assets.** For a single person, this is all countable assets minus $2,000. For a married couple, subtract the amount the nursing home spouse can exclude ($2,000) and also subtract the CSRA

($154,140 in the "100% states"; 50% of the total countable assets of both spouses in the other states, but never more than $154,140).

Calculate the **net monthly expenses ("A")** of (i) single person (nursing home cost + other living expenses – total income) or (ii) married couple (nursing home cost + other living expenses of both spouses – total income of couple).

To find the divisor figure for your state, go to:

https://www.medicaidplanningassistance.org/penalty-period-divisor/

Divide the **total amount of countable assets** by the total of the **net monthly expenses ("A")** plus the **penalty divisor ("B")**. This will give you the total number of months penalty you will be facing.

So far we have this:

Amount available ÷ (A + B) = # of months penalty.

Multiply the **number of months penalty ("C")** by the **penalty divisor ("B")**. This will give you the amount of the gift you can make: **C x B = gift amount.**

To see how the numbers work in several sample cases, see **Case Studies** in Chapter 17.

Why the Classic Half-a-Loaf Method No longer Works

Unfortunately, the method described above will no longer work for gifts made on or after the date of enactment of the DRA, i.e., February 8, 2006. The new DRA rule states that a penalty period on a gift will not start to run until the Medicaid applicant actually applies for Medicaid and would have qualified for Medicaid *but for the gift penalty*. As a result, if a person makes a gift of half of his or her assets and retains the "other half," the penalty period will not even start to run until those retained assets are spent down, because until that time, the applicant has too many assets to qualify for Medicaid. In other words, if Roland gives away $50,000 and retains $52,000, under the old rules the penalty period (10 months) starts to run on the date he makes the gift. He could then use the money he retained to pay privately for those 10 months, and then apply for Medicaid after the penalty period has expired, when he's down to his $2,000 exclusion amount.

But under the new rules, if Roland keeps $52,000 in the bank, even if he applies for Medicaid now, the penalty period will not start to run until he has spent down to $2,000 and applies again, i.e., in 10 months. At that point, since he would no longer have any assets (other than the $2,000 exclusion amount), he would qualify for Medicaid *but for the gift penalty.* Unfortunately, his $50,000 gift falls within the 5-year lookback period, so Roland, who at this point now has only $2,000, is faced with a 10-month penalty. Clearly he cannot pay privately for the next 10 months with the amount of money he has left. Thus, his family will wind up paying for him, using the $50,000 he gave them 10 months ago. At the end of the penalty period, his entire $100,000 will have been spent on his nursing home care, leaving his family with nothing. He's no better off than had he made no gifts at all.

New Half-a-Loaf Alternative Methods

There must be a better way! Well, there are several alternatives that take the new law into consideration. Let's take a look at them, now.

Gift + Return of Half the Assets (Reverse Half-a-Loaf)

The simplest solution is for the Medicaid applicant to make the gift of all the excess assets, apply for Medicaid, and be turned down because of the gift. This starts the penalty period running. Then, the recipient(s) of the gift simply return "half" the assets back to the Medicaid applicant. This reduces the penalty period to half as long as initially imposed, and the applicant now has sufficient assets to pay privately for the penalty period. Note that the word "half" is in quotes: it rarely works out that the amount to transfer is exactly 50% of the amount of excess assets. You will need to follow the formula set out above to come up with the exact amounts to use.

The way it works in practice is that the applicant makes the gift and applies for Medicaid. The state calculates a penalty period based on this original gift. Each month the recipient of the gift returns a portion of the original gift to the applicant, which, when combined with the applicant's other income, is sufficient to pay the nursing home bill at its private rate.

Eventually the point will be reached when the continually reduced penalty period equals the amount of time that has passed since the date of the original gift. Assuming the calculations were correctly made, the applicant should at this point have disposed of the entire original gifted amount (by a combination of the balance of the original gifted amount and the returned amounts that were spent on care), leaving the applicant with sufficiently low assets to qualify for Medicaid.

When that point is reached, the state agency is notified, and the applicant documents the amount of the returned payments. That justifies a reduced penalty period, which has by this time expired, so the applicant should now qualify for Medicaid.

In some states a second application must be made, but in others eligibility will be granted following verification that the recalculated penalty period has expired.

The important consideration with this approach is that not all states permit the recipient of a gift to return less than the entire amount of the gift received (known as a "partial cure") as a way of reducing the penalty. If your state is such an "all or nothing" state, then this technique is simply not available to you. However, some states actually allow a person to count separate gifts (e.g., to different children) separately for purposes of the "all" requirement. Under this rule, so long as each separate gift is completely reversed, the penalty period can be reduced; the recipients do not have to reverse *all* the separate gifts to eliminate or reduce the penalty.

Gift + Annuity

By combining an outright gift to family members and a purchase of a Medicaid annuity with the balance of the countable assets, half-a-loaf planning can still be done. Here is how it works.

Example:

After Roland has calculated how much he should give to his children and how much he needs to retain in order to cover the resulting penalty period, he purchases a "Medicaid annuity" from an insurance company familiar with the Medicaid annuity rules. So if he had determined he needed to keep $50,000, then he purchases an annuity worth $50,000 and applies for Medicaid to start the penalty period. Since a Medicaid annuity is not counted as a resource, it's as if Roland has no money, so he would qualify, *but for the gift*. As a result, the penalty period will start running immediately. Of course, he still must pay privately for the penalty period, since Medicaid will not cover him during this period. That's where the annuity comes in: each month the annuity company sends him a check, which he uses to pay his nursing home bill. The term of the annuity should always equal the penalty period.

NOTE: After making the above calculations, be careful that the annuity payments are not so high that the Medicaid applicant won't qualify for Medicaid, based on having too much income! See *The "Too Much Income" Problem*, immediately below.

Gift + Promissory Note

An alternative to the Gift + Annuity technique is the Gift + Promissory Note technique. The calculations are exactly the same, except that instead of having the Medicaid applicant use the excess funds to purchase an annuity, he or she loans those funds to a family member. In exchange for the loaned money, the family member signs a "Promissory Note" agreeing to pay back the loaned money over a specified time period (i.e., the number of months equal to the penalty period). According to the terms of the Note, each month a payment is made to the Medicaid applicant, who will then use that money to cover the nursing home expenses. As described in detail above the loan must be documented in writing, all payments must be equal in amount, and the note must prohibit cancellation upon the lender's death.

NOTE: After making the above calculations, be careful that the Note payments are not so high that the Medicaid applicant won't qualify for Medicaid, based on having too much income! See the discussion below, *The "Too Much Income" Problem.*

The "Too Much Income" Problem

Whether utilizing an annuity purchase or a loan and Promissory Note combination, if the payments will be made to the Medicaid applicant, there is a possible trap to be aware of: since the payments of the annuity or Note each month are treated as "income" for Medicaid eligibility purposes, it is possible for the payments to be so high that the Medicaid applicant will have *too much income* to qualify for Medicaid. Not all states have this rule, but if they do, then it means that the penalty period will *not* start running at the time of the gift and will only start running after the payments from the annuity or Note are completed! That would be a disaster, because the Medicaid applicant will have no assets at that point, and yet be ineligible for Medicaid. Once again, the family members who received the gift money will have to turn around and use that money to pay the nursing home during the penalty period, leaving them nothing at the end.

To avoid this problem, the payments must be set so that they do not cause the Medicaid applicant's income—both his or her own income, such as from pension and Social Security *and* the annuity or Note income—to exceed the maximum income permitted by the state's rules. The family members who received the gift money will have to dip into those funds to cover the shortfall between the actual costs of the nursing home and the total permitted income of the Medicaid applicant. Coming up with the optimal amount of money to be gifted, while calculating the size of each payment, can be extremely complicated, with numerous interrelated moving parts, and will typically involve setting up a complex spreadsheet to work all this out. So do not be surprised by the legal bill to come up with the correct numbers: it is definitely not a trivial or easy task!

Gift of Interest in Home + Sale of Balance

As discussed above, an individual's home is an excluded asset (assuming the equity is under $713,000). However, upon the death of an individual who was covered by Medicaid, the state will want to be repaid for the Medicaid expenditures it made on behalf of that individual. The longer the owner has been in the nursing home, the greater the debt to the state. It's possible that it will take the entire value of the house to pay back the state.

How can the owner of the house, in this situation, preserve the greatest amount of value of the house, and still qualify for Medicaid in the shortest period of time? If the owner does nothing, he can qualify for Medicaid immediately, but then following his death Medicaid estate recovery against the house will eliminate any of the benefits he initially received from Medicaid. If he sells the house before applying for Medicaid, he will be over-resourced and will be faced with a long spenddown period.

One approach to protect at least part of the value of the home is as follows:

> Owner of the home (who is in the nursing home) transfers 50% of the home to a child (or an irrevocable trust). Then owner applies for Medicaid. If owner has no other countable assets, owner will be eligible for Medicaid but for the gift of the interest in the home. Therefore, the penalty period will start running. Once the penalty is determined, the house can be sold. This will generate enough cash for owner to pay privately during the penalty period. Thus, 50% of the home's value has been protected. (Again, the actual percentage to be gifted away must be calculated by running through the half-a-loaf formula set forth above.)
>
> Note, however, that you must consider how long houses for sale are sitting on the market. If the applicant has no other cash with which to pay the nursing home during the ensuing penalty period, and the house is not selling, the nursing home will want to be paid by someone. If the house will sell shortly, the recipient of the gifted interest in the home (e.g., the trust or child) can pay the nursing home during the pre-sale

period. If the transfer is to a trust, however, there will have to be cash in there already for this to work. And if houses are sitting a long time, this technique may just not be workable.

Compare this to selling the home first, then making the gift and applying for Medicaid: in such case, since the Medicaid applicant will be sitting there with cash equal to half the proceeds of the house sale, applying for Medicaid will not start the penalty period running. That's because with all that cash, the applicant will not be Medicaid eligible *but for the gift* (the requirement to get the penalty period started). As a result, the applicant will have to go the additional step of using those proceeds to purchase an annuity or lend money to family members in exchange for a Promissory Note. Transferring the interest in the house first, then applying for Medicaid, and then selling the house, avoids those complications.

If the home has increased in value significantly since its purchase, exposing a sale of the home to capital gains tax, the option of transferring the gifted portion of the house to a trust rather than outright to children will make more sense. In this case, the trust will be drafted as a so-called irrevocable "grantor trust." Such a trust reserves certain powers to the homeowner even after the interest is transferred to the trust, with the result that the homeowner is deemed the owner of the entire house for income tax purposes. The result of this technique is that upon the later sale of the house, the full $250,000 capital gains exclusion may be used. If the interest in the home had instead simply been gifted to one or more children, then the amount of taxes attributable to the gifted portion would *not* be eligible for this exclusion.

What if the homeowner still has some extra cash to spend down? A variation on the above is to transfer that cash *plus* a percentage interest in the home to children, apply for Medicaid, and then sell the home to obtain the cash to pay privately during the penalty period. Once again, the actual percentage to be gifted away must be calculated by running through the half-a-loaf formula set forth above, this time including both the cash and the value of the house in the gifted portion.

Exceptions

The following transfers are exceptions to the general rule that penalizes gifts made by a person applying for Medicaid.

Although these exceptions eliminate gift treatment for Medicaid purposes, they do not affect the possible *gift tax* cost of such a transfer. For the transfers to trusts, it is recommended that the trust give a "limited power of appointment" to the grantor of the trust, which will eliminate any possible gift tax. In addition, there is no gift tax that applies to outright gifts between spouses.

Transfer to Spouse

A transfer between spouses is never penalized. After all, the assets of both spouses are added together when one spouse applies for Medicaid. Since it does not matter whose name the assets are titled in when the "snapshot" is taken, there is no reason to penalize a transfer of assets between spouses. Hence, it is a good idea to title all assets in the name of the Community Spouse as soon as it looks likely that the other spouse will be requiring nursing home care within a relatively short period of time.

Trust for the Sole Benefit of the Spouse

A transfer of assets by the Medicaid applicant to a trust for the "sole benefit" of the Community Spouse will not result in a penalty period. The spouse must be the sole beneficiary of the trust and payments must be made to or for the benefit of the spouse on a basis that is "actuarially sound" based on the spouse's life expectancy. One way to do that is to have distributions based on the same table that governs minimum distributions to a beneficiary of an IRA. Because a trust established by one spouse is deemed established by *either* spouse, such a trust is treated as if the Community Spouse set up the trust for him- or herself; under the trust rules discussed in Chapter 9 the entire amount of the trust would still be countable as the Community Spouse's own assets, should the Community Spouse ever need to apply for Medicaid also. Thus, the only reason for setting up such a trust is if the nursing home spouse wanted to limit the amounts that could be distributed to or for the benefit of the Community

Spouse each year. Such limitations on distributions might be useful if the Community Spouse, for example, was not a good money manager or might easily be talked into foolish expenditures.

Transfer to Blind or Disabled Child

A transfer of assets to the Medicaid applicant's child who is legally blind or who is disabled as determined by Social Security rules (e.g., the child is receiving SSDI), will not result in a penalty period. However, if the child is disabled, be careful that the transferred assets do not cause the *child* to lose his or her government benefits as a result of the gift! The best way to make the gift yet protect the child's government benefits is to make the transfer into a trust for the child (see next paragraph).

Trust for the Sole Benefit of a Blind or Disabled Child

A transfer of assets by the Medicaid applicant to an irrevocable trust for the "sole benefit" of the applicant's blind or disabled child will not result in a penalty period. The child must be the sole beneficiary of the trust and payments must be made to or for the benefit of the child on a basis that is "actuarially sound" based on the child's life expectancy; one way to do that is to have distributions based on the same table that governs minimum distributions to a beneficiary of an IRA. Again, be careful that the transferred assets do not cause the *child* to lose his or her government benefits as a result of the gift! The trust must be set up as a "supplemental needs trust" by your attorney.

Upon the beneficiary's death, the balance of the trust will *not* have to be used to repay the state for any Medicaid outlays it made on behalf of the trust beneficiary. However, if the beneficiary dies before his or her normal life expectancy, leaving assets in the trust, those assets will be payable to the beneficiary's estate, where they will be subject to estate recovery (however, there is no estate recovery for benefits—other than nursing home care—that were provided to an individual under age 55). Alternatively, if the trust includes a provision to pay back the state for any Medicaid benefits it paid out on behalf of the beneficiary during his or her lifetime, then the trust does *not* have to pay out actuarially and it *can* provide for additional beneficiaries upon the initial beneficiary's death (after satisfying the state's claim).

Trust for Sole Benefit of a Disabled Person Under Age 65

A transfer of assets by the Medicaid applicant to an irrevocable trust for the "sole benefit" of a disabled individual (other than him- or herself) under age 65 will not result in a penalty period. This exception is not limited to trusts for children, so it could be for the use of a disabled grandchild, sibling, or other family member. The disabled individual must be the sole beneficiary of the trust and payments must be made to or for the benefit of the individual on a basis that is "actuarially sound" based on the individual's life expectancy. Once again, the trust must be worded carefully so that the transferred assets do not cause the disabled individual you are benefiting to lose his or her government benefits as a result of the gift.

Upon the beneficiary's death, the balance of the trust will *not* have to be used to repay the state for any Medicaid outlays it made on behalf of the trust beneficiary. However, if the beneficiary dies before his normal life expectancy, leaving assets in the trust, those assets will be payable to the beneficiary's estate, where they will be subject to estate recovery (however, there is no estate recovery for benefits—other than nursing home care—that were provided to an individual under age 55). Alternatively, if the trust includes a provision to pay back the state for any Medicaid benefits it paid out on behalf of the beneficiary during his or her lifetime, then the trust does *not* have to pay out actuarially and it *can* provide for additional beneficiaries upon the initial beneficiary's death (after satisfying the state's claim).

Transfer of the Home: Caretaker Child

A transfer of the home to the Medicaid applicant's child (of any age) will incur no penalty, if the child was living in the house *for at least two years* immediately prior to the date the parent was admitted to the nursing home, and the child provided care to the parent prior to the parent entering the nursing home that permitted the parent to delay entering the nursing home. The parent's home must be the child's sole residence during this period. The child will need to document (i) that the parent would have needed to move into a nursing home but for the child's assistance (a physician's assessment will be needed for this), and (ii) what the child actually did for the parent during this two-year period (keep good records!). Here is what one state requires from a child seeking to utilize this exemption:

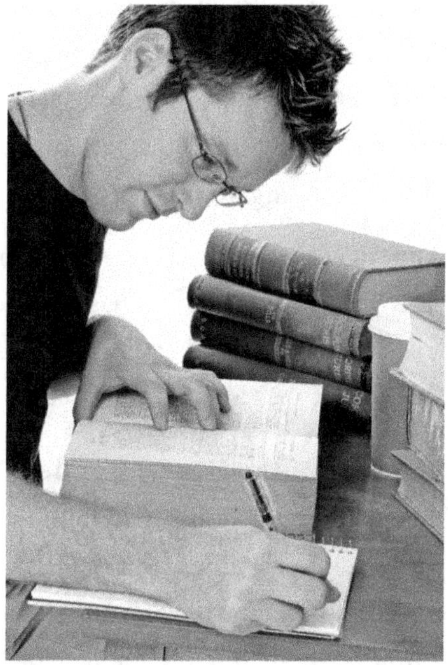

1. a written statement from the parent's primary physician describing the type and amount of care provided by the child and the effect such care may have had on the parent's ability to reside in the home;
2. written documentation regarding the medical condition of the parent;
3. copies of either: documentation from the Dept. of Social Services, canceled checks, bank statements, income tax forms or other documents showing that the child provided care and/or financial support to the parent; and
4. copies of the child's income tax returns for the prior three years or bank statements or bills in the child's name showing the parent's residence as the child's residence from two years prior to the date of the parent's entry into the nursing home and to the present date.

If the parent will need to be admitted into a nursing home before the child has cared for the parent for the full two years, then the parent will not be able to take advantage of the caretaker child exception. Also, if the child lives with the parent for over two years, but then moves out before the parent goes to a nursing home, this exception will not work: the two-or-more-year-period that the child takes care of the parent must immediately precede the parent's entry into the nursing home.

Although the federal statute does not explicitly deal with this, to be on the safe side, wait until the parent has entered the nursing home before making the transfer to the caretaker child. Until then, you won't know for certain whether you've met the two-year requirement.

Transfer of the Home: Resident Sibling

A transfer of the home to a sibling of the Medicaid applicant will incur no penalty, if the sibling has an equity interest in the home and was living in the house *for at least one year* immediately prior to the date the applicant was admitted to the nursing home. Note that care is not an issue, as it is with the "caretaker child" exception above.

Having an "equity interest" in the home means that the brother or sister must already own some percentage interest in the home at the time the balance of the home is gifted to him or her. The owner can deed a tiny percentage (1%) to the sibling who will be living there, but then should preferably wait at least one year before entering the nursing home in order to take advantage of this exception.

It would be safer to wait until after the owner has entered the nursing home before making the transfer to the sibling. Until then, you won't know for certain whether the sibling has met the one-year requirement.

Transfer of the Home: Minor, Blind or Disabled Child

A transfer of the home to a child of the Medicaid applicant who is under age 21, blind, or disabled will incur no penalty.

Transfers Exclusively for Non-Medicaid Purposes

If you can prove that you made a gift purely for a purpose *other than* Medicaid planning, then even if the gift falls within the lookback period, it will be ignored.

You must present to the state convincing and objective evidence proving that the assets were transferred *exclusively* for a purpose other than to qualify or remain eligible for Medicaid. Transfers to avoid the Medicaid lien or estate recovery are included in the definition of Medicaid eligibility.

There is a rebuttable presumption that the transfers were made for purposes of Medicaid eligibility. In other words, if there was *any* expectation of applying for Medicaid that could reasonably be inferred to be a factor in your decision to transfer the asset, the presumption cannot be successfully rebutted. Merely stating that you were ignorant of the transfer penalty or verbal assurances that you were not considering Medicaid eligibility when the transfer was made are not sufficient. Nor can you rebut the presumption by stating that the transfers were done "for estate planning" or "for probate avoidance" purposes.

If the amount of your assets (and those of your spouse, if you are married) remaining after the transfer are sufficient to pay for medical (including long-term care) and living expenses reasonably expected to be incurred for you or your spouse for the next five years, then you should be able to claim that you certainly did *not* make the transfer for Medicaid planning purposes. After all, you had plenty of money to self-pay!

As to gifts you have not yet made, if you make gifts to, say, your grandchildren for their college education, or you buy a car for one of your children, or even make a large charitable donation, and at the time you're in good health and have sufficient assets to cover any possible long-term care for the next five years, you should document all of this at the time you make the gift. This information may come in handy should the unexpected happen and you or your spouse winds up applying for Medicaid within five years of the gift.

Hardship Waiver

Under the federal Medicaid laws enacted in 2006, either the facility *or* the resident may petition the local Medicaid office for a hearing, to waive the imposition of the penalty from the earlier gifts made by the resident. The penalty period *may* be waived if:

- ④ the individual is unable to obtain medical care without the receipt of Medicaid benefits,
- ④ the gifted assets have been irretrievably lost and all reasonable avenues of legal recourse to regain possession of them have been exhausted, and
- ④ application of the transfer penalty would deprive the individual of medical care such that the individual's health or life would be endangered or would deprive the individual of food, clothing, shelter or other necessities of life.

Assuming that relocating the nursing home resident back to his or her home would put the resident's life in jeopardy (since there may well be no one there to properly care for the resident), it should not be difficult to prove that the penalty from the prior gifts should be waived. That being said, the states are making it exceedingly difficult for anyone to take advantage of the hardship waiver without great effort and a perfect set of facts.

As you can see, the above procedures will put the resident and his or her entire family in a very precarious situation and cause much emotional turmoil for several months, while this whole thing is sorted out. Meanwhile, the family will have to incur significant legal fees to represent the resident in the hearing to waive the penalty. Accordingly, this is not something you would want to plan for!

Nursing Home Eviction Rules

If a nursing home resident has made gifts to family members, runs out of money after residing for some period of time in a nursing home, and a hardship waiver cannot be obtained, federal law permits the nursing home to evict the resident for non-payment, *if* the nursing home does all of the following:

- Prepares a summary of the resident's mental and physical health status
- Prepares a post-discharge plan of care for the resident which will assist the resident to adjust to his or her new living environment; and
- Notifies the resident and a family member or legal representative of the resident of the pending discharge at least 30 days in advance of the discharge, letting them know of the resident's right to appeal the discharge action to the state.

The point of the above is that nursing home residents *can* be evicted from the facility for non-payment of their monthly fees. Accordingly, it is vital that the Medicaid rules be understood and followed, and appropriate appeals taken, in order to avoid this harsh result.

Transfers to Community Spouse

Since there is never a penalty for transfers between spouses, as a general rule a married couple should arrange to title as much of their assets as possible in the name of the Community Spouse, as soon as possible. Here are the reasons to do so:

- Once the CSRA is determined, any additional assets required to increase the Community Spouse up to that amount *must* be transferred from the nursing home spouse to the Community Spouse within one year of the Medicaid eligibility starting date.
- Should the nursing home spouse become incapacitated, it may be impossible to implement some of the techniques discussed in this book. For example, it may be possible to protect a substantial portion of the Community Spouse's assets even if the Community Spouse should die before the nursing home spouse. Such planning is not possible, however, if those assets are still in the name of the incapacitated nursing home spouse at the death of the Community Spouse.

Purchase Long-Term Care Insurance, Make Gift

If you are able to qualify for long-term care insurance, consider purchasing a policy that has at most a five-year coverage option. Once the insurance is in place, make a gift of the maximum amount of assets you can afford to part with, considering your ongoing expenses and current income. If you need nursing home care within the five years, then you will have your bills covered by the policy and won't have to worry about the gift penalty. Once five years from the date of your gift has passed, you will be able to apply for Medicaid, since the prior gift is now outside of the lookback period. Thus, the most you'll ever have to pay the long-term care premiums is for five years. If possible, purchase a policy with decreasing coverage: in year 1 (the year you make the gift), you need coverage for five years; when you renew the policy in year 2, only for four years; in year 3, only for three years, etc. That way, you are not paying for more coverage than you need, because starting in year 6 you will be able to qualify for Medicaid, and you won't need the long-term care insurance coverage anymore.

If you already have long-term care insurance, be sure to take that into consideration when determining how much money you can give away. If you have a policy that gives you full and complete coverage for five years, then you can make as large a gift as you wish to, since even if you have a stroke the next day and have to move into a nursing home, your long-term care insurance will cover you during the five-year lookback period. Upon the termination of the coverage of your insurance policy, you can apply for Medicaid, since the lookback period no longer includes the gifts you made more than five years ago.

What if you only have three-year coverage? Then you can still make a large gift, but you'll have to consider how you will pay privately for the two-year "gap" between the period covered by your insurance and the five-year lookback period.

Example:

Martha currently owns a long-term care policy that will pay for her nursing home care for up to three years. That means that if Martha has to move into a nursing home, the policy will pay her bills there for no more than three years. Since Martha's health is currently pretty good, she decides to make a large gift of her assets to her three children. However, she is careful to retain sufficient assets in her own name to cover the cost of the nursing home for the two-year period between when the insurance runs out and the lookback period no longer can count her gift. In other words, if Martha makes the gift and the next day has to go to the nursing home, her long-term care insurance policy will pay her bills there for the next three years. At the end of the three years she cannot apply for Medicaid, because that would cause a very long penalty period. Accordingly, she's set aside enough assets in her own name to cover the cost of a nursing home for a two-year period. This only matters if she enters the nursing home within the first two years, and with each passing month, that's one month fewer that she may have to pay for out of her own pocket.

Of course, it's possible that after two years Martha has not entered the nursing home. Since her three-year policy will now take her to the end of the lookback period, she does not have to worry about retaining assets to cover her care privately. So now she needs to dispose of the excess assets that she had set aside for the potential two-year gap. To avoid this problem, she could have given *all* her assets to her children, with the understanding (although not legally binding) that the children would pay for their mother's care if indeed she needed to enter the nursing home within the first two years.

Disclaiming an Inheritance

If a relative dies and leaves you (or your spouse) an inheritance, usually that's good news. But what if you're already on Medicaid? Assuming all your needs are being taken care of in the nursing home by Medicaid, that money won't do you any good and will only disqualify you from the Medicaid program. You'd then have to spend down the inheritance till it's gone, and then reapply for Medicaid once you're broke. So much for the benefit of the inheritance!

Under state law, you can "disclaim" an inheritance or gift under a person's will, which means you refuse to accept the asset or money left to you. As a result, you're treated as if you never got the asset or money and it passes to the person next in line: if it was an inheritance (i.e., your relative died with no will), then it passes according to state law; if it was left to you under a will or trust, then it passes according to the terms of the will or trust. In most cases, it will pass to your children. In any event, the person making the disclaimer has no power over where the disclaimed money goes.

Unfortunately, the general rule is that for Medicaid purposes, the disclaimer is looked at as if you *did* receive the money and then turned around and gave it away. As a result, you'll be faced with a penalty for that gift.

Accordingly, the disclaimer won't accomplish what you hoped it would. In most cases, it's best if you accept the inheritance/gift, and then deal with it the same as any other countable asset, using one or more of the many techniques and options discussed in this book.

But what if you're incapacitated at the time you receive the inheritance? In that case, hopefully you will have signed a comprehensive durable power of attorney before you became incapacitated, one that specifically authorizes gifting to family members for Medicaid planning. If no gifting clause is in the power of attorney document, it still may be possible to convert at least some of the assets into non-countable resources, as described above (see *Converting Countable Assets to Non-Countable*, Chapter 10). If no durable power of attorney is in existence, then the family members may have to petition the local court for permission to make such gifts, assuming such court-authorized gifting is even allowed by state law.

Chapter 15

POST-ELIGIBILITY ISSUES

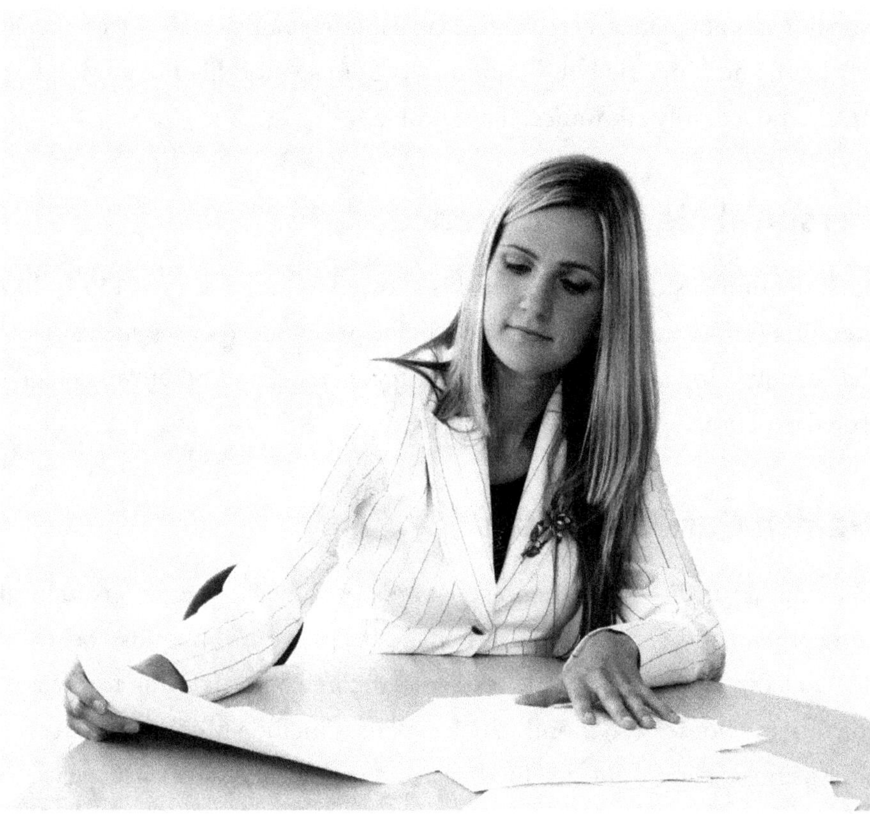

Patient's Share-of-Costs

Once the nursing home resident has been approved for Medicaid, the state will pay the entire nursing home bill at the state reimbursement rate, less the resident's "share-of-costs" amount. The monthly share-of-costs amount would be the resident's income (from Social Security, pension, etc.), reduced by the personal needs allowance, certain medical expenses not covered by Medicaid (see below), and if married, the Community Spouse monthly income allowance ("MIA") and a family allowance, if applicable.

Personal Needs Allowance

A nursing home resident on Medicaid is allowed to keep between $30 and $200 (depending on the state) or so per month, for personal expenses such as barber/beauty shop appointments, clothing, toiletries, and other miscellaneous personal expenses.

Health Care Expenses

Medical and remedial care expenses that are not subject to being repaid by an outside organization (such as a health insurance program) may also be deducted from the nursing home resident's income before paying the balance to the nursing home each month. Such expenses include Medicare and other health insurance premiums, deductibles, and coinsurance and necessary medical or remedial care recognized under state law but not otherwise covered under the state Medicaid program, subject to reasonable limits the state may establish on the amount of these expenses.

This is sometimes referred to as Post-Eligibility Treatment of Income (PETI). It would cover, for example, a hearing aid that was lost, and for which Medicare would not cover a replacement. The nursing home resident can put in a request with the state to have this expense covered out of the resident's own income. Assuming the request is approved, it would allow the resident to pay for the hearing aid instead of paying that money to the nursing home.

In essence, Medicaid is paying for the hearing aid by permitting the resident to shift income from the nursing home to the hearing aid company.

Even nursing home expenses incurred before the date of Medicaid eligibility may be considered "medical expenses" and therefore covered by this provision. This should be comforting for the nursing home patient who did not apply for Medicaid as soon as he or she should have. For example, say the nursing home has not been paid for a few months and then the nursing home patient finally applies for Medicaid. As discussed in Chapter 4 ("Retroactive Coverage"), it is possible in most states to apply for coverage for up to three months prior to the date of application, *if* the applicant would have qualified at such time, had he or she applied. But if the patient would not have qualified at such time due to having too much money or other reasons, or if the bills go back further than three months, at least the nursing home can be paid out of the patient's income once the patient is approved for Medicaid coverage.

Post-Eligibility Transfers by the Community Spouse

There is a split among the states on the treatment of transfers made by the Community Spouse *after* the nursing home spouse is determined to be eligible for Medicaid. Some states allow the Community Spouse to make such transfers without affecting the nursing home spouse's eligibility for Medicaid, but others treat it as if made by the nursing home spouse, thereby causing a period of disqualification. Often they make a distinction between a transfer of the house and that of other assets. Thus, you'll need to check with an experienced elder law attorney in your state to find out the current rule that applies to you, if you are thinking of doing such transfers. Of course, any such transfers will affect the Medicaid eligibility of the Community Spouse should he or she apply for Medicaid him- or herself after making such gifts, but that's a different question than if such gifts affect the eligibility of the *nursing home spouse.*

If the Community Spouse Dies First

If the Community Spouse dies before the nursing home spouse, the risk is that the assets owned by the Community Spouse will pass into the name of the nursing home spouse, causing the nursing home spouse to become immediately ineligible for Medicaid until the inherited assets are spent down. This often happens because the Community Spouse assumes he or she will outlive the nursing home spouse and never gives this any thought. Typically, the wills of the husband and wife leave everything to each other, if living, otherwise to the children. If they never had wills, then their state law would generally do the same thing, awarding all the assets to the surviving spouse. Accordingly, when the Community Spouse dies, all the assets that were protected as the CSRA are now handed over to the nursing home spouse, who of course has no use for them.

So what should the nursing home spouse do if the Community Spouse dies first, leaving all of his or her assets to the nursing home spouse? As discussed above, the nursing home spouse cannot simply "disclaim" (refuse) the inheritance or gift under the will. That will be treated as if the spouse received the assets and then made a penalty-causing gift of those assets. Instead, the best alternative in most cases is for the surviving spouse to accept the inheritance or gift under the will and then deal with the assets using one or more of the techniques discussed in this book.

However, to avoid this problem, the Community Spouse should create a new will, one that takes this problem into consideration.

Elective Share Problem

The first reaction of most people is to say, "*Well, why can't I just omit my spouse from my will entirely?*" While this can certainly be done, it will not be effective, because the laws of every state grant a surviving spouse certain minimum rights to the assets of the deceased spouse. The reason for this is to prevent a spouse from creating a will that leaves nothing to the surviving spouse, leaving that spouse impoverished and a ward of the state.

Each state has its own scheme to accomplish this by guaranteeing a surviving spouse some percentage of the deceased spouse's estate. This is called a spouse's "elective share" or "statutory share." The amount of the elective share depends on the laws of the state the couple resides in. Some states give a surviving spouse a one-third interest in the deceased spouse's estate no matter how long they were married. Other states use a gradually increasing percentage, e.g., 10% if married for under 2 years, 20% if between 2 and 4 years, 30% if between 4 and 6 years, etc., with a maximum of 50% if married 10 or more years.

If the Community Spouse tries to defeat the elective share by making gifts to children or other relatives, these gifts can be brought back into the calculation, depending on how long ago they were made and whether or not the other spouse consented to the gift. Some states apply the elective share to a so-called "augmented estate." This is an extremely complex set of rules that determines exactly which assets of the first spouse to die are subject to the elective share. In some cases, even assets that were given away years ago are brought back into this calculation, as are certain transfers to trusts. Just think of the last bald probate attorney you met—it's because he tore his hair out trying to figure out the elective share and augmented estate statutes!

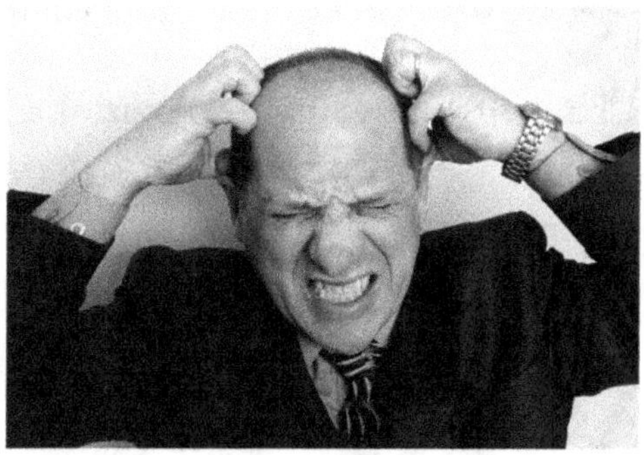

Assuming that the Community Spouse will not have completely depleted his or her estate by death, a conservative approach, then, would be for the Community Spouse to write a new will, one that leaves *only the minimum amount necessary to satisfy the elective share* outright to the surviving (nursing home) spouse. The balance can safely be left to the children or other relatives. As you can see, this will give the spouse only half or a third (depending on the state law), immediately saving the other half or two-thirds of the assets from having to be spent down on nursing home care. This simple change can easily save thousands of dollars for the other family members!

The problem with the outright gift under the will is that not only does it cause the immediate disqualification of the surviving spouse from Medicaid benefits, but it exposes the full amount of the elective share to estate recovery, as assets of the surviving spouse. If the surviving spouse dies shortly after receiving the money, then most if not all of that money will wind up being paid over to the state under the estate recovery program, as reimbursement for its Medicaid payments.

A better approach is to leave the elective share amount in the form of a trust that satisfies the elective share statute yet will not be included in the surviving spouse's estate. The success of this approach depends not only on how the state permits the elective share to be structured, but also on how it handles estate recovery: some states limit recovery only to the probate estate, some go further. Again, this must be determined by an experienced elder law attorney in your state who can assist your travel through these very complicated waters!

The main point of the above is that it is not enough to qualify one spouse for Medicaid, without planning for the possibility that the Community Spouse may die first. Be sure that as part of your Medicaid planning your elder law attorney prepares a new will for the Community Spouse, one that deals with the "elective share problem" discussed in this section.

Change Beneficiary Designations

As discussed above, it is vital for the Community Spouse to change his or her will. But don't forget about investments that pass by beneficiary designation and *not* by will! This includes IRAs, 401(k)s, life insurance policies, and annuities. If any of these were retained as part of the Community Spouse's CSRA, be sure to change the beneficiary designation so it does not go directly to the nursing home spouse. Whether any of these need to fund the elective share trust discussed above or not is a difficult calculation that can only be determined by your elder law attorney, due to the variations in state law that affect the calculation of the elective share.

Divorce Option

One option that may be considered in order to protect the assets of the Community Spouse is a divorce. Often a couple is understandably reluctant to go this route, because of the social stigma of a divorce. However, if a spouse has Alzheimer's, advanced dementia, or other life-restricting illness, the undeniable fact may be that the couple's life together is already over, as a practical matter. A divorce at this point is not due to any lack of love between the two spouses but is purely for the financial protection of the Community Spouse; the nursing home spouse will be well-cared for via Medicaid payments. But without a divorce the Community Spouse's assets may be reduced to the point that the long-term welfare of the Community Spouse can be put in jeopardy.

That being said, some states may not allow a divorce from an incapacitated spouse. If they do, they probably will not permit all assets to be awarded to the Community Spouse. The general rule is that there must be an "equitable distribution" of the assets and income of the couple. The circumstances and needs of each spouse must be considered. If all the assets are awarded to the Community Spouse, the state Medicaid department could view that as a gift from the nursing home spouse, causing a period of ineligibility. However, if it is demonstrated that the nursing home spouse's bills will be well-covered by Medicaid, but the living expenses of the Community Spouse are not financed by government programs, there should be a good argument for awarding a greater percentage of the assets to the Community Spouse.

As you can see, you will need a good divorce attorney who must be guided by an experienced elder law attorney, to make this work! However, in the long run, it could positively affect the financial well-being of the Community Spouse without affecting the overall level of care of the nursing home spouse.

Post-Gift Transfers by Children

If you are going to make gifts to more than one child, it would be a good idea for the children to do one of the following after they receive the funds, assuming the plan is for the money to be kept available for your benefit should the need arise:

(A.) **The children open up a joint bank account.** Once the children receive the gift, they can make equal contributions of the funds you gave them into a joint bank account. It's important for them to document who contributed what, so that if one of the children is sued or divorced or goes bankrupt, only that child's share of the bank account can be attached by the creditor or divorcing spouse. In most cases, the account should be set up so that all contributing children must sign off on withdrawals, to protect against a child who falls on hard times (or temptation) and dips into the funds for personal use without telling the siblings. The advantage of this arrangement is that the money is segregated from the children's other assets, so they are more likely to use it for the parent's benefit, should the need arise. The disadvantage is, what if one of the children dies or becomes incapacitated? Who will succeed to the child's interest in the bank account? And will the surviving children go along with continuing to leave the deceased child's interest in that bank account? One partial solution would be to have each child sign a limited power of attorney to the other children, authorizing them to access the bank account if one of the children becomes incapacitated.

(B.) **The children create a joint trust.** For even greater protection, once the children receive your gift, they can make equal contributions of the money you gave them into a single trust. One or more children can act as trustee although having an independent (i.e., non-family member) trustee will both better insulate the money from creditors of the children and hopefully avoid family squabbles on use of the funds. The trust can name you as beneficiary, to cover any of your "supplemental needs" (i.e., expenses *not* paid for by Medicaid, once you are eligible). This guarantees that the money will be available for you, should you ever need it, since it is now out of the children's names completely. Also, if a child is sued, divorced, or goes bankrupt, the share of your money you gave them is protected.

> Alternatively, the trust can allow distributions to be made *only* back to the children, who could then turn around and use it for your benefit, similar to the joint account arrangement discussed above. The advantage to this alternative is that it makes it much harder for the state to claim that the trust was "really" established by and for the parents, causing inclusion of the trust property in the parents' countable assets.

If the children are going to set up such a trust, it is important that they do *not* hire the same attorney who assisted you with your Medicaid planning. Also, the children should allow a reasonable amount of time to pass before they create and fund this trust. What's "reasonable"? Unfortunately, there is no hard and fast rule; clearly a week is too soon and five years longer than necessary, so pick somewhere in between! The attorney the children hire is in the best position to advise them about this issue. The reason for the above precautions is to make sure that the children's funding a trust for you is an independent act of theirs and not part of a coordinated plan that you and the children agreed to in advance of your gifts to them. Otherwise, the state Medicaid authorities can argue that in essence, *you* set up the trust *for yourself*, using your own money, and therefore all the assets in the trust are now countable under the self-funded trust rules!

Moving from State to State

What happens if you or your family member must move from one state to another and then apply for Medicaid? What if you or your family member is already in the Medicaid program and then moves? Will you lose your eligibility?

First of all, it is a violation of the U.S. Constitution to impose a residency requirement on an individual who moves into a state and then needs to apply for Medicaid. So the day after you move you can apply for Medicaid.

That being said, you still need to meet the asset and income requirements discussed throughout this book. So if the requirements for eligibility are different in new State B than they were in old State A, you must meet the eligibility requirements of the new state before Medicaid will cover you.

Example:

Joe lives in State A, where his wife, Josephine, has her nursing home costs paid by Medicaid. Joe deeds his house to his children to avoid estate recovery in the event he should die before his wife and also to avoid having the house in his name should he ever require nursing home care. Under the laws of State A, such transfer of the house by the Community Spouse does not impact the eligibility of the nursing home spouse.

In order to be nearer their children, Joe and Josephine move to State B. Unfortunately, State B treats a gift of the residence by the Community Spouse as a disqualifying transfer affecting the Medicaid eligibility of the nursing home spouse, so after the move, Josephine will be disqualified from receiving Medicaid payments for many months if not years! Had they remained in State A, all her nursing home bills would have continued to have been paid under that state's Medicaid program.

As you can see, even if you were already on Medicaid in State A, there is no guarantee that you will qualify for Medicaid in State B. Even if you must move, it would be advantageous to understand the rules of the new state, so that you don't make any gifts or implement any planning techniques in the old state that may have negative consequences in the new state. By understanding the rules of both states, you may be able to adjust your timing of gifts before the move, as well as the timing of your Medicaid application in the new state.

In addition, because many states operate under federal waiver programs, the relocated individual may have to go on a long waiting list to get Medicaid coverage, and indeed the coverage under the prior state's waiver program may simply not be available in the new state (for example, some states cover assisted living costs and some do not). Again, once you move, you are governed by the program rules and coverage of the new state.

Bottom Line: If you have the option to move or not, you would be wise to check with an experienced elder law attorney in the state you are considering moving to. Be sure you understand how the rules of the new state would apply to your situation, so you won't be faced with any nasty (and expensive) surprises!

Chapter 16

ESTATE RECOVERY

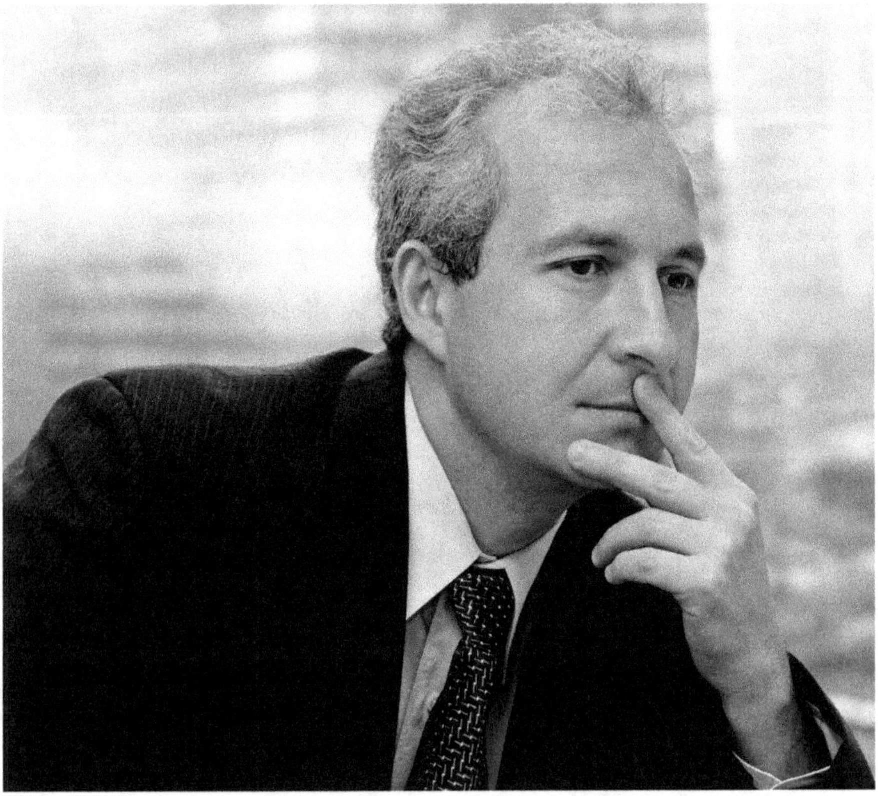

Upon the death of any individual who was covered by Medicaid while institutionalized (or a non-institutionalized Medicaid recipient who was at least age 55 at the time of receiving benefits), the state must seek to recover all of the expenditures it made on behalf of the now-deceased Medicaid recipient for nursing home costs, medical costs (hospital and prescription drugs) while in the nursing home, Medicare premiums and co-payments during this time, and HCBS payments. To be clear, regarding a non-institutionalized Medicaid recipient, the state can only recoup for benefits paid after the recipient was at least age 55.

Since this recovery is not made until after the death of the recipient, it is known as "estate recovery."

In essence, while you thought you had qualified for a government benefit, all you've really received is an interest-free loan! And upon your death, the government wants its loan paid back.

Prior to 1993, such estate recovery was optional—a state could implement it or not. However, in that year a new federal law was passed (known as OBRA '93) that mandated that every state *must* seek estate recovery from its Medicaid-receiving residents following their deaths. While some states managed to delay implementation of this federally mandated law until just recently, by now every state finally has a recovery statute in place.

Now if you're sharp, you may be thinking "Wait a minute… if someone qualifies for Medicaid, they have to be essentially broke. So where exactly is this money coming from to repay the state?" That's a good question, and the good news is that if your family member died owning nothing, then indeed the state is out of luck. It can't go after the kids' money. It can't go after a surviving Community Spouse's money. There must be some assets that the nursing home resident had a legal interest in, at the time of death, in order for the state to be repaid. That legal interest is defined as the "estate" of the deceased Medicaid recipient. However, how the word "estate" is defined varies from state to state, thereby affecting what assets the particular state can recover against.

Definition of "Estate"

All states must seek recovery at least from the "probate estate" of the Medicaid recipient. This is typically defined to include only assets that would pass by will. Such definition includes assets titled in the sole name of the decedent, but excludes assets that pass by beneficiary designation (such as a life insurance policy, annuity, IRA, 401(k), or similar plan payable to someone other than the insured's estate); POD (pay on death) bank accounts; TOD (transfer on death) stock certificates or brokerage accounts; trust property; joint bank accounts; and jointly owned real estate or other property that passes by operation of law automatically to the surviving owner(s) by right of survivorship.

Expanded Definition of "Estate"

Under the federal law, any state may adopt an expanded definition of "estate," to include any one or more of the following: assets conveyed to a survivor, heir or assign of the deceased individual through joint tenancy, tenancy in common, survivorship, life estate, living trust, or other arrangement (such as an annuity). In other words, the definition of "estate" could now include virtually any asset in which the deceased nursing home resident had any legal interest the moment before death. Currently, only 13 states actually limit estate recovery to probate assets, with the other states adopting various degrees of the maximum permitted by federal law. It is important that you know exactly what is and what is not subject to estate recovery in your particular state, so that you may plan accordingly.

Planning for Change

Unfortunately, even if you reside in a state that does not currently use an expanded definition of "estate," there is no guarantee that it may not do so at some time in the near future. Worse, a recent case held that there is no "grandfathering" for Medicaid recipients when the law changes midway through their nursing home stay: whatever law is in effect upon the death of a

Medicaid recipient will apply, even if that means that assets that were not subject to recovery earlier in the recipient's nursing home stay are subject to recovery at the time of his or her death. This is another reason for only working with an elder law attorney who is not only active in his or her field and keeps up with legislation that may be introduced in your state affecting estate recovery, but who is also aware of trends in other states that may affect future legislation in your state. Of course, there is always the possibility that laws may change, and no attorney has a crystal ball, but you increase your odds of doing the best possible planning by working with a "plugged-in" and savvy elder law attorney.

Exceptions

There are some exceptions that prevent estate recovery.

If you were under age 55 at the time you received Medicaid benefits *other than nursing home care*, then you will be exempt from estate recovery *for the amount of those benefits.*

No recovery may be made against a Medicaid recipient's estate until after the death of the surviving spouse, if any, and only at a time when there is no surviving child of the recipient who is under age 21 or a child of the recipient who is blind or totally and permanently disabled.

Note that it is not necessary that these individuals be living in the recipient's home for these exceptions to apply. Nor is it necessary that the estate—or any part of it—be left to any of these individuals in order for the ban on recovery to apply.

Estate recovery against your home will also be prevented (or postponed) if a lien has been imposed on your home and a child or sibling of yours is living in the home, in certain circumstances discussed in more detail below.

If all else fails, there's an exception to estate recovery if such recovery would work an "undue hardship" on the surviving family members. One example would be where the excluded asset is a working farm, and a forced sale of that farm would throw surviving family members out of work.

Timing of the Recovery Claim

Technically, the federal law states that recovery can be made "only after the death of the individual's surviving spouse." So if, for example, the at-home spouse dies a month after the Medicaid recipient spouse, a state *could* file a claim for recovery at that time. Many states, however, have taken a more liberal reading of this, and so long as there *is* a surviving spouse, no recovery will be made, no matter how long or short the surviving spouse lives. You'll need to check your own state's laws to find out which rule applies to your situation.

Notwithstanding the above, even in a state where recovery may be made after the surviving spouse's death, there typically is an additional limitation that applies to *all* claims against an estate: all states have a statute of limitations that bars claims against an estate that are made more than a certain number of months after the death. In many states, that limit is one year. So, in a state with such a law, if the surviving spouse dies more than a year after the Medicaid recipient spouse, it will be too late for the state Medicaid recovery unit to file its claim for estate recovery. Some states have gotten around this limitation by filing the claim within the limitations period, but delaying recovery until after the death of the surviving spouse. Other states simply exempt the state's claims from the statute of limitations and allow the state to file a claim against the probate estate even after the normal limitations period has expired.

If a state can only file a claim when there is no child under 21, can it wait until the child attains age 21 and then file its recovery claim? Once again, this must happen within the statute of limitations period, assuming there's not a blanket exemption if there's a surviving child under age 21.

Procedure and Time Limit

As discussed above, if recovery is limited to the "probate estate," then the law of most states requires the state to file a timely claim against the estate, just as any other creditor of the decedent must do.

If a lien was filed against the house, however, the state may have a longer time in which to satisfy its claim. Exactly *how* much longer depends on the lien law of your state; again, you would need to check with an elder law attorney in your state, but be prepared for the attorney not knowing the answer right off the bat, since this is an unsettled question in many states.

Sometimes the family of a deceased Medicaid recipient will attempt the "lay low" approach, not opening a probate estate and hoping that the limitations period will expire before the state files its claim. If that happens, then the family will indeed "win," since at that point it will be too late for the state to collect its money from the estate. However, many states have now implemented procedures where they are notified of the death of anyone in a nursing home who was a Medicaid recipient, and if probate of the estate is not opened by the family within 30 days, the state itself—as a creditor—may petition the court to open the estate, and then file its claim for estate recovery.

Waivers

In certain limited circumstances, the state must refrain from seeking recovery against the estate if it would result in undue hardship. For example, a disabled family member may be living in the deceased Medicaid recipient's home, and it would be deemed a hardship if there were a forced sale of the house, rendering the family member homeless.

In addition, a state may waive recovery if it is not cost-effective, i.e., the value of the house (or the amount to be recovered) is small in relation to the administrative cost of seeking recovery.

Married Couples' Issues

In planning for estate recovery for a married couple, one must consider the possibility that either spouse may be the survivor.

If the Nursing Home Spouse Dies First

Following the death of the nursing home spouse, the state is limited to recovering assets in which the nursing home spouse had a legal interest at the time of death. However, if there is a surviving spouse, federal law bars the state from filing for estate recovery until after the surviving spouse dies. The states are divided among those that completely waive estate recovery if there is a surviving spouse, those that merely defer enforcement of the claim until the later death of the spouse, and those that use a combination approach. In any event, the state can never go after assets that were always owned solely by the surviving Community Spouse.

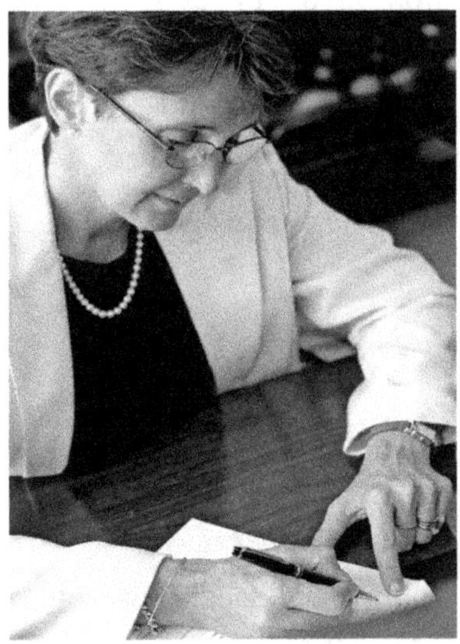

As a general rule, the state can only go after assets in the deceased nursing home spouse's "estate" by filing a claim against that estate. Under the expanded definition of "estate" however, assets that pass to someone else immediately upon the death of the nursing home spouse may still be subject to recovery. How can the state identify those interests?

A few states have begun to apply a "tracing" approach, whereby assets that once belonged to the nursing home spouse and that passed into the name of the Community Spouse at the death of the nursing home spouse (whether by will, right of survivorship, etc.) can be reached by the estate recovery rules after the death of the Community Spouse.

If the Community Spouse Dies First

If the Community Spouse predeceases the nursing home spouse, the big issue is what happens to the assets owned by the Community Spouse upon his or her death. The last thing you want to have happen is for the assets to pass to the surviving spouse, who is in the nursing home on Medicaid. If that happens, the nursing home spouse will be immediately disqualified from receiving Medicaid, by virtue of being "over resourced," and any of those inherited assets still in the surviving spouse's name at his or her death will be subject to estate recovery. Accordingly, this possibility must be carefully planned for, because you never know which spouse may die first.

Avoiding Estate Recovery

As discussed above, merely qualifying for Medicaid is not enough if upon the Medicaid recipient's death the state can file a claim against the property of the deceased recipient, demanding to be repaid every dime of benefits it paid out on behalf of the recipient. However, there are some planning techniques that you can implement to minimize or eliminate the state's right of recovery.

Eliminate Probate Assets

First of all, in the 28 states where estate recovery is only made by a claim against the probate estate of the Medicaid recipient (so-called "probate estate only" states), all you need be sure of is that the Medicaid recipient has *no* probate estate at death.

For example, you can title an automobile in joint names with a child. You don't even have to have a driver's license to be an owner of a car. So the car would be titled as "Mary Smith and John Smith, JTWROS." John is Mary's son, and upon Mary's death, sole title to the car passes automatically to him outside of probate. "JTWROS" stands for "joint tenants with right of survivorship." (Be sure to check your state's motor vehicle titling rules to be sure this will work in your state!) Since one car of any value is excluded during Mary's lifetime, it's protected during her life and escapes estate recovery on her death.

The same approach can even be taken for her house. Since a Medicaid recipient's house is normally excluded during her lifetime (up to $713,000 in equity value), it's only at the recipient's death that there's a problem. So to avoid the house being included in Mary's probate estate, she can title her house as JTRWOS with her son John, on her deed. CAUTION: Adding another person's name to the deed is a gift of an interest in the house, effective upon the date of the deed! Thus, when Mary has her attorney add her son John's name to the deed, she has just made a gift of 50% of the house to him. Although gift tax is rarely an issue, it should be considered. More importantly, though, is that this is a Medicaid-disqualifying transfer, with a large penalty attached. If Mary wants to go this route, she may be unable to apply for Medicaid for *five years* after she signs the deed.

Also, what if John is sued or divorced or goes bankrupt? Mary may still think of the entire house as "hers," but the creditor or divorcing spouse will view that 50% interest in the house as an asset of John's, and it could be subject to attack. Mary may find herself out on the street if the house has to be sold to satisfy the judgment or divorce settlement.

Some states permit adding another person to a deed while giving them less than 50%. Ideally, you would want to give your child as small a percentage interest in the house as possible, yet still have the house pass to the child upon your death via the right of survivorship. For example, a 1% joint interest would reduce the amount of the gift as well as expose less of your house to the child's creditors. However, sometimes the rule for real estate law purposes differs from the rule for Medicaid purposes. So, a word to the wise: be sure that the attorney who is doing the new deed for you is up-to-date on the effect that will have on your Medicaid eligibility!

Sell House, Do "Half-a-Loaf" Gifting

It is also possible to remove the house from the Medicaid recipient's estate by *selling* the house and structuring a type of "half-a-loaf" transfer with the proceeds (you make a gift to other family members and retain just enough of the proceeds to carry you through the resulting penalty period).

Since the transferor/owner already was on Medicaid, this would only make sense if the amount of additional private pay payments the transfer will cause will be less than the amount of possible estate recovery. Thus, the longer you are on Medicaid, the more likely it is for this technique to save the family any money. You may want to calculate the number of months of disqualification based on the half-a-loaf formula discussed above and wait until your debt to the state (based on the private pay rate LESS the patient pay amount) exceeds the number of months of disqualification (resulting from the gift) x the private pay rate.

Transfer House Shortly Before Death

If the Medicaid recipient—or other family member if the recipient is incapacitated—transfers the home shortly before death, the home will no longer be part of the deceased Medicaid recipient's estate, and thus will escape recovery.

Such a transfer will cause the imposition of a period of ineligibility, requiring the family to pay privately for the nursing home care during this period.

However, this may be a small price to pay to avoid the much larger bill of estate recovery.

Example:

Mildred, a widow, is nearing the end of her life. She has been in the nursing home for five years, on Medicaid. During this time Medicaid has paid the nursing home approximately $285,000 on her behalf. If Mildred died today, the state would seek reimbursement from her estate for this amount, for which it would look to her house, her only asset. Instead, her family deeds the house to themselves using a durable power of attorney that specifically authorizes such gifting, and the family dutifully reports the gift to the state. Because of this gift, she is immediately disqualified from Medicaid and her family must now pay for her final months in the nursing home. Upon Mildred's death, she no longer owns the home, leaving nothing for the state to attach in satisfaction of its estate recovery claim. Of course, if the state had already filed a lien against the house (see below), then this technique would not work.

Some states may claim that such a transfer of the home is a **"fraudulent transfer."** A "fraudulent transfer" is a transfer of property by a person for the purpose of defeating, hindering, or delaying the person's creditors. If a state were successful in making such a claim, all it would mean is that the house would have to be retransferred to the Medicaid applicant and once again would be subject to estate recovery. The family would be no worse off than it would have been had it done nothing. Unlike actual "fraud" against the state (such as hiding assets and not reporting them to the state on a Medicaid application), which can result in criminal or civil penalties, a "fraudulent transfer" carries no such penalties. There is a strong legal argument that the fraudulent transfer rules do not apply to transfers in a Medicaid context, since there are already specific federal statutes within the Medicaid sections that set forth the penalties for gifts, which would trump the fraudulent transfer rules. Needless to say, you should consult with an attorney before doing anything like this.

Liens

To prevent Medicaid recipients from disposing of their assets prior to death, thereby avoiding the state's attempt at estate recovery, states are permitted to file "liens" against certain property of a Medicaid recipient.

A lien (pronounced "lean") against your home is a recorded document filed by a creditor of yours that prohibits the sale of your home without first satisfying the existing debt. It is similar to a mortgage, which prohibits you from selling your house without first paying off the bank. In the Medicaid context, it is filed by the state to guarantee repayment of all the money it will pay out for your care while you are on the Medicaid program.

Under the Tax Equity and Fiscal Responsibility Act of 1982 (known as "TEFRA"), states have the option of imposing liens to ensure repayment of their Medicaid expenditures. Thus, the state you live in may or may not impose liens.

When Applied

Following notice and opportunity for a hearing, a lien may be placed on the home of the Medicaid recipient once it is established that the recipient is not expected to return to his or her home. Note that this should not be confused with the continued exclusion of the home, no matter how likely it is as a practical matter that the Medicaid recipient will ever return home, so long as the "intent to return home" is maintained. In other words, the state can determine that you are both *unlikely* ever to return to your home for TEFRA lien purposes and *likely* to return home for Medicaid eligibility purposes!

The lien may be filed no matter how old you are, so long as you are receiving Medicaid for nursing home or home and community based services (HCBS). Recovery may only be made after the death of the Medicaid recipient or, if sooner, upon the sale of the home.

Exceptions

The lien may not be *imposed* at the time any of the following are lawfully residing in your home:

④ your spouse
④ a child of yours who is under age 21
④ a child of yours who is permanently blind or disabled, as defined under the Social Security regulations
④ a brother or sister of yours who has an equity interest in your house and who has lived there at least one year prior to your entering the nursing home.

The lien may not be *enforced* if any of the following are lawfully residing in your home and *have been* lawfully residing in your home since the date you entered the nursing home:

- ④ a child of yours who lived there at least two years prior to your entering the nursing home and whose care allowed you to delay your going there; or
- ④ a brother or sister of yours (who may or may not have an equity interest in your house) who has lived there at least one year prior to your entering the nursing home.

Finally, the lien must be removed if you leave the nursing home and actually move back home.

Chapter 17

CASE STUDIES

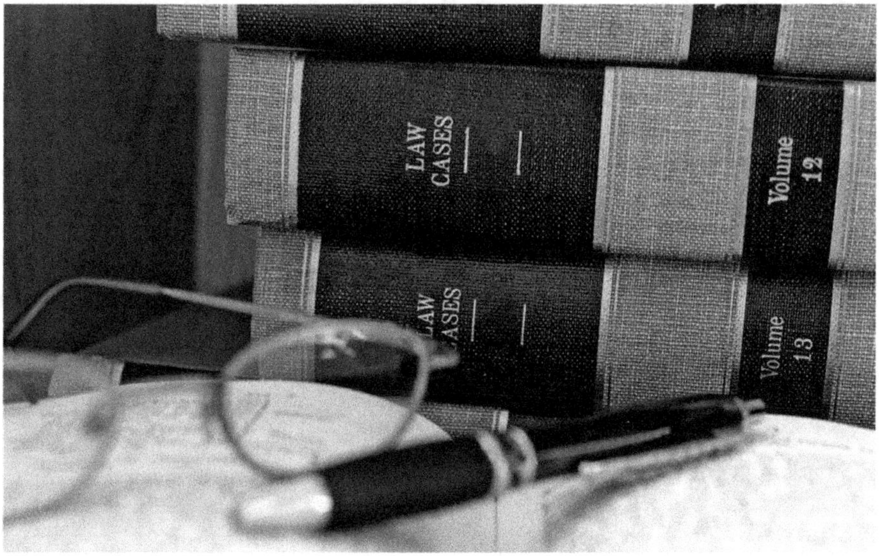

The following are "case studies," or examples of the thinking that a sharp elder law attorney would go through in analyzing the issues of actual clients and coming up with realistic solutions. Going through them will help you synthesize and learn how to apply many of the various techniques discussed in this book.

Summary of Case Studies

- ④ **Study #1**

  Single person already in the nursing home, with assets of $215,000, no home, and income of $2,090/month. Discusses use of half-a-loaf planning with a Medicaid annuity.

- ④ **Study #2**

  Single person already in the nursing home, with assets of $42,000, a home, and income of $900/month. Discusses various options for protecting the home from estate recovery, as well as spenddown techniques.

- ④ **Study #3**

  Married couple with one spouse already in the nursing home, with assets of $300,000, a home, and income of $2,500/month. Discusses CSRA calculation, spenddown options, half-a-loaf gifting, and how to protect the home from estate recovery.

- ④ **Study #4**

  Married couple with neither spouse in the nursing home, with assets of $950,000, a home, and income of $9,000/month. One disabled child. Discusses use of an irrevocable trust, funding a Supplemental Needs Trust for the disabled child, and transferring the home to their disabled child or to her trust.

- ④ **Study #5**

  Single person not in the nursing home, with assets of $300,000, no home, and income of $1,600/month. Discusses use of an irrevocable trust, half-a-loaf planning with a Medicaid annuity, and the interaction of these two techniques depending on when, if ever, the person will enter a nursing home.

Study #1:

Single Person with $215,000 in assets, no home, and $2,090 monthly income.

George is single and has the following assets:

CDs	$100,000
Bank accounts	5,000
IRAs	110,000
2010 auto (Kelley Blue Book value)	12,000

Here is his monthly income:

Social Security	$990
Federal retirement pension	1,100
CD interest	250

His monthly expenses:

Nursing home fee	$5,500
Health insurance premiums	200
Miscellaneous (haircuts, toiletries, magazines, etc.)	100

Let's go through this step-by-step.

- ④ **Total Assets.** The auto is excluded, so we don't count it for this purpose. That leaves a total of $215,000 of countable assets. He is allowed a personal exclusion of $2,000, so the amount he must "spend down" is $213,000.
- ④ **Net Monthly Expenses.** The total of his typical monthly expenses is $5,800. From this we subtract his income. We don't count his investment

income of $250 for this purpose since the assets that generate this income will be depleted soon, so his countable income is $2,090 per month. Thus, his monthly out-of-pocket expenses come to $5,800 - $2,090 = $3,710. In other words, he has to dip into his savings each month to cover this shortfall of $3,710.

④ **First Thoughts.** Since George is already in the nursing home, his planning options are somewhat limited. He cannot make gifts and wait five years until the expiration of the lookback period; that would be too expensive. However, he can always reduce his countable assets by making gifts to family members using the half-a-loaf technique and then buying a Medicaid annuity with his remaining funds. That would allow him to qualify for Medicaid much sooner. So let's take a look at how to calculate that.

④ **Penalty Divisor.** After checking with his state Medicaid office, he finds out that his state's penalty divisor is $5,000.

④ **Calculating the Proper Size of Gift.** Dividing the total amount of George's countable assets ($213,000) by the total of his net monthly expenses ($3,710) + the penalty divisor ($5,000) gives us this:

$213,000 ÷ (3,710 + 5,000) = $213,000 ÷ 8,710 = 24.45,

or approximately 24.5 months penalty.

Multiply the above number of months penalty (24.5) x the penalty divisor ($5,000) = $122,500. Thus, **he should make a gift of $122,500 and use the balance of his assets ($90,500) to purchase a Medicaid-friendly annuity.**

George must immediately apply for Medicaid. Although he now only has countable assets of $2,000, he has just made a large disqualifying gift, so he will be denied Medicaid coverage. However, it is necessary to apply at this point in order to get the penalty period running.

Assume the annuity will pay George $3,710 per month for the 24.5-month period. The annuity, combined with his Social Security and pension income, will be sufficient to cover his nursing home bill during the penalty period. Upon the expiration of the 24.5-month penalty period, the annuity payments stop, and George can now re-apply for Medicaid. Because the penalty period will have expired by then, he will immediately qualify for Medicaid.

NOTE on Income Cap Rules: In some states, George's total income ($5,800) will be too high for him to qualify for Medicaid without him funneling his income through a "Miller Trust" (see discussion in Chapter 6). Even then it may *still* be too high for him to qualify for Medicaid. And it is important for George to be able to qualify for Medicaid *but for the penalty-causing gift*, in order to start the penalty period running. In such case, the amount of the annuity will have to be adjusted so that the monthly payments to George cause his total income to be just under the maximum "income cap" amount. Since that will not give him enough money each month to cover his nursing home cost, his family will have to dip into the money he already gave them to cover this shortfall during the penalty period. As you can see, these calculations have a lot of moving parts, and they *must* be made by an experienced elder law attorney if this approach is to be successful.

Proof:

If George decides to make this gift of $122,500, he will have $90,500 to use for buying a Medicaid annuity. The annuity will pay him $3,710 per month. His cost of living for the 24.5-month penalty period (above what he can cover with his income) will be $3,710 per month x 24.5 = $90,895. That leaves him with an excess of $395. Undoubtedly the nursing home costs will increase over the two-year period when he will be paying privately, so it's doubtful he will have too much money at the end of the period.

Result:

By making this gift, George has protected over $122,000 for his family, while qualifying for Medicaid sooner.

NOTE: His Social Security and pension income will continue to be paid to the nursing home even after he is on Medicaid. The Medicaid program will simply pick up the difference between these income payments and the actual nursing home costs.

What if George is Not Yet in the Nursing Home?

As you can see from the above example, once George is in the nursing home, any gift has a penalty period that results in George having to pay out of his own pocket until the penalty period expires. Even though George saved over $122,000, he still had to spend over $90,000 of his money before he qualified for Medicaid. If he had made the gift earlier, he could have protected it *all* for his family.

So let's assume that George is not yet in the nursing home, but wants to plan ahead. Assume his assets and income are the same. The only difference will be his monthly living expenses. Since he's living at home, he won't have the nursing home bills, but he will certainly have grocery and restaurant expenses, he may be driving his car, and he may even need to hire part-time assistance as his health worsens. Unfortunately, this calculation forces George to guess how many months he will remain at home, not needing to move to the nursing home. If he makes a larger gift and needs to go to the nursing home sooner than anticipated, then his family will have to use some of the gifted assets for his care. If he remains in better health than he thought, then he may have money left over at the end of the penalty period. Such calculations are at best an educated guess, based on George's expected health and financial needs. However, it is almost always better to come close than to do nothing! Once again, the assistance of an experienced elder law attorney is absolutely necessary to guide the family through all of these options.

Dealing with the Auto

As discussed above in the Estate Recovery section, merely qualifying for Medicaid is not the end of the story, if there are any excluded assets owned by the Medicaid recipient at the time of his or her death. In George's case, planning must also be done to protect George's auto against estate recovery, keeping in mind the extent of the state's ability to reach George's "estate" following his death.

George can simply retitle his auto into joint names with one of his children. Also, if he will not need the auto anymore, he can give it to one of his children. In either case, he is making a gift. However, since the auto was an excluded asset, there is no penalty: there is never a penalty for gifting an excluded asset (other than the home).

Study #2:

Single person with $42,000 in assets, a home, and $900 monthly income.

Maria is single and has the following assets:

Bank accounts/CDs	$42,000
Home	250,000
2001 auto (Kelley Blue Book value)	12,000

Here is her monthly income:

Social Security	$900

Her monthly expenses:

Nursing home fee	$5,500
Health insurance premiums	200
Miscellaneous (haircuts, toiletries, magazines, etc.)	100

Let's go through this step-by-step.

- ④ **Total Assets.** The home and auto are excluded, so we don't count them for this purpose. That leaves a total of $42,000 of countable assets. She's allowed to keep up to $2,000 as her personal exclusion, so really her "spenddown" amount is actually $40,000.
- ④ **Net Monthly Expenses.** Adding up her typical monthly expenses, the total is $5,800. From this we subtract her income. Thus, her monthly out-of-pocket expenses come to $5,800 - $900 = $4,900. Clearly, she cannot afford the nursing home without outside help, be it from Medicaid or family.
- ④ **Medicaid Eligibility.** Without doing any planning, Maria's remaining savings will be completely gone in a little over 8 months. At that point, she should immediately qualify for Medicaid coverage of her nursing home bills. Maria's Social Security income will continue to be paid to the nursing home even after she is on Medicaid. The Medicaid program will simply pick up the difference between her income and the nursing home cost.
- ④ **First Thoughts.** Although Maria does not have a lot of savings, there is no reason to just spend it until it's gone. With relatively small amounts of countable cash, setting up a half-a-loaf strategy may not be cost-effective, because of the complexity and legal fees involved. Instead, she should try to spend down her extra $40,000 by the following:

    - improve her house
    - upgrade her auto
    - pre-pay her own funeral and burial expenses
    - pre-pay burial spaces for other family members

    If there is still any money left after the above, she can certainly utilize the half-a-loaf method to gift half of that balance and use a promissory note or Medicaid annuity for the other half. Alternatively, Maria can retain the balance of her savings to pay privately for a few months, and then apply for Medicaid coverage. Sometimes that will help her move up closer to the top of the waiting list for the nursing home and secure placement sooner.

④ **Estate Recovery.** As far as Maria is concerned, getting herself placed in an excellent nursing home should be her top priority. She cannot afford to reside in a facility that does not accept Medicaid payments unless she is willing to sell her house to cover those costs (which could easily exceed the entire value of her house in a few years). Fortunately, there are many excellent facilities that accept both private pay and Medicaid. So if Maria does Medicaid planning or not, her situation really will not be that much different.

On the other hand, her family will lose not just $40,000 if Maria does no planning, but thousands more due to estate recovery upon her death. Let's assume the Medicaid reimbursement rate for her nursing home is $4,000/month. Her Social Security will pay part of that, leaving a net cost of $3,100/month. So if she lives for another five years after her money runs out, her estate will owe the government 60 months x $3,100 = $186,000. In order to pay that back to the state, the house will have to be sold, with just a portion of the full value of the house passing on to the family. As you can see, Maria's family really has more at stake than she does, so avoiding estate recovery should become the main focus of any Medicaid plan for Maria.

Since the only asset Maria will possess at her death is her home, let's take a look at some of the options of avoiding estate recovery against her home.

Possible Solutions

1. **Gift House Five Years in Advance.** At least five years before Maria thinks she may need nursing home care, she deeds the house to her children. She can continue to live in the house, with the permission of her children. Since the lookback period is five years, so long as she does not apply for Medicaid before that date the gift will be ignored. Upon her death, since she no longer owns the house, it is protected against estate recovery.
   This could be risky, though: what if one of the children gets sued or divorced or goes bankrupt? A child's interest in the house can then be

reached by these creditors, possibly forcing a sale. If Maria no longer has legal ownership, she could wind up on the street.

2. **Gift Joint Interest in House.** Maria can add one or more children onto her deed, ensuring that each owner is a "joint tenant with right of survivorship" or "JTWROS." That form of ownership ensures that upon Maria's death, her interest evaporates and avoids estate recovery (unless she lives in a state with an expanded definition of "estate"). She still must wait out the five-year lookback period, though. Another disadvantage is that she is a co-owner of the house with the children, so she cannot sell it without their permission and if they are sued or divorced or go bankrupt, the child's interest in the house could be attached, once again possibly causing her to lose her ability to live in her home.

   In some states, it is possible to have unequal joint tenancy interests. If such is the case, then a tiny percentage interest can be given away, such as 1%, causing a very small gift (see *Gift Value*, Chapter 11). Then, when Maria applies for Medicaid, she will only be faced with less than a month's penalty. Her children would certainly be willing to pay that cost, in exchange for her protecting the entire value of the house by virtue of the joint ownership deed.

3. **Transfer House to Trust.** Maria can also transfer the house into an irrevocable trust. The advantage is that she can continue to control the house, possibly even serve as her own trustee, yet protect it against creditors of her children. There can be no estate recovery against the trust, since Maria gave up ownership in the house on the date she deeded it into the trust. She can retain a right to live in the house for her lifetime, by putting that requirement right into the trust document. That can actually be useful for income tax purposes, since it will cause the basis of the house to be re-adjusted to the value on Maria's date of death; that can save the children capital gains taxes when they go to sell the house after Maria's death. Once again, though, Maria may have to wait out the five-year lookback period before applying for Medicaid.

4. **Gift House, Retain Life Estate.** To protect Maria's right to continue to live in her house as long as she is able, and to protect it against creditors of her children, she can deed just a "remainder interest" in the house to her children (or to an irrevocable trust). Another way to think of this type of deed is that she is giving the house to her children (or the trust) but retaining a "life estate" in the house; that's what protects her lifetime interest to live in the house. On her death, there can be no estate recovery against the house (unless she lives in a state with an expanded definition of "estate" that includes life estates).
5. **Sell House, Move in with Child.** If Maria thinks that she may need to move into a nursing home before five years but after at least one year, Maria can sell her home and purchase an interest in the home of one of her children. She can structure this either as a purchase of a life estate in the child's home or a purchase of a joint interest.

    - **Purchase of Life Estate.** Maria can purchase a life estate in the child's home. By looking up her age in the life estate table, she can calculate the percentage of the child's home she needs to buy for her $250,000 to avoid making a gift to the child. So if Maria is age 80, her life estate is worth 0.43659 (43.659%) according to the table. If she has $250,000 to invest in the child's house, then she can purchase a life estate in a house worth $572,620 ($250,000 ÷ 0.43659).

      Of course, the chances of her child's house being worth exactly that amount are extremely unlikely. If the child's house is worth less than that, Maria will be making a gift to the child who owns the house if she gives the child $250,000. That is because at age 80, her life estate is worth 43.659% of the value of whatever house she owns a life estate in. So if the $250,000 is worth more than 43.659% of the value of the entire house, she's paying more for her life estate than she needs to. For example, if the child's house is only worth $400,000, she only needs to pay the child 43.659% of $400,000, or

$174,636, for a life estate in the entire home. If she pays $250,000 for that life estate, she's essentially overpaying by $75,364; that amount is a gift to the child. If she did that, she'd have to wait five years to avoid a penalty on the amount of that gift. On the other hand, if the house is worth more than $572,620, then she will be buying a life estate in less than 100% of the house; in that case, it's easy for the deed to adjust for that.

In any case, upon her death, her interest terminates, leaving the home once again titled 100% in the name of the child (or child and child's spouse, if that's how the house was formerly titled).

NOTE: If Maria does not live in the house for at least one year after she signs the deed, then her purchase of the life estate will be deemed to be a gift to her child of the entire $250,000, for Medicaid purposes. Thus, this should only be done if she feels fairly certain, based on her current health, that she will not need nursing home care for at least one year.

- **Purchase of Joint Interest.** To avoid the requirement that Maria live in her child's home for at least one year in order to avoid having the purchase treated as a gift, she can instead purchase a joint interest in the child's home. If the child's home is valued at, say, $500,000, Maria can purchase a 50% joint interest (with a right of survivorship) in the child's home and move in. Since Maria is paying her child the fair market value of a 50% interest in the home, it's not a gift, so there's no penalty period to worry about. After a reasonable period of time, should Maria need to go to a nursing home, her interest in her child's home will be an excluded asset. Although there is no "one year requirement" for the joint purchase, clearly the longer she is there, the better. Upon her death, the interest passes to the child under the deed, by operation of law, and there is no estate recovery against the house (unless

Maria lives in a state that has an expanded definition of "estate" that includes joint property).

6. **Effect of Lien.** If Maria lives in a state that allows for the filing of a lien against the house of a Medicaid recipient, the general rule going back hundreds of years (the so-called "common law" of the United States) is that the lien on a person's joint property interest is extinguished when that person dies and the right of survivorship passes to the other joint owner(s). So if Maria has changed the title on her house—or moved into a child's house—so that it is now owned by her and her child as joint tenants with right of survivorship, the state will ordinarily be out of luck trying to enforce its lien to collect estate recovery against the property after Maria's death, since the house will then be owned 100% by the child. However, to be on the safe side, Maria should check with an attorney in her state to see if a specific statute was passed that overrules the common law rule just stated. Certainly if Maria has given all interests in the house away (either outright to her children or to an irrevocable trust) and does not own any interest in the house at her death, no lien can attach to it. But if she does any of the other options discussed above, there is the possibility that the lien may take precedence over any joint owner's interest, at her death.
7. **Crisis Planning.** If Maria is already in the nursing home and has done no planning with the house, is she out of luck?

   If she lives in a state where a small percentage joint tenancy gift can be made, that's probably her best bet.

   Otherwise, she will probably have to sell the house and do some of the other techniques discussed in this book, such as half-a-loaf gifting, etc. She should definitely consider the *Gift to Trust of Interest in Home + Sale of Balance* technique discussed in Chapter 14.

   If she does nothing, many states have a law that permits a "lien" to be placed on the house after six months. The lien prevents the house from being sold unless the state is first reimbursed for its Medicaid payments on Maria's behalf. If that happens, then the family will have to face up to repaying the state for Maria's Medicaid coverage, after her death. The family will either keep her home and pay off the state (whereupon it will file a Release of Lien) or sell the home and pay back the state. In any event, if Maria's estate recovery bill *exceeds* the value of the house, the family is *not liable* for the shortfall.

Study #3:

Married Couple with $300,000 in assets, a home, and $2,500 monthly income: CRISIS PLANNING!

Mark and Isabelle are married. Isabelle recently moved into a nursing home, and Mark continues to live in the family home.

Here are their combined assets:

Bank accounts and CDs	$10,000	W*
IRA	100,000	H
Variable annuity	50,000	H
Mutual funds	140,000	JT
Home	250,000	JT
2010 auto (Kelley Blue Book value)	12,000	W

*Owned by husband (H), wife (W), or jointly (JT)

Their monthly income:

Social Security	$900	W
Social Security	1,200	H
Pension	400	H

Their monthly expenses:

Nursing home fee for Isabelle	$5,500
Health insurance premiums	200
Miscellaneous (haircuts, toiletries, magazines, etc.)	100
Upkeep of house (average)	600
Food for Mark	350

Let's go through this step-by-step.

④ **Total Assets.** The home and auto are excluded, so we don't count them for this purpose. Everything else is added up, regardless of whose name it is titled in: husband's, wife's or joint. Thus they have $300,000 in countable assets.

④ **Net Monthly Expenses.** The couple's typical monthly expenses total $6,750. From this we subtract their combined income of $2,500. As you can see, they are short $4,250 each month. At this rate, this couple will be completely broke in less than four years if they do nothing. A better idea is to do some Medicaid planning!

④ **Medicaid Eligibility**

- **Assets.** Assume they live in a "100% state." Since the value of the couple's combined assets exceeds the CSRA ($154,140), that is the maximum amount Mark will be allowed to keep; the balance of their assets, other than Isabelle's $2,000 personal exclusion, will have to be spent down or otherwise depleted before Medicaid will pay Isabelle's nursing home bills. Thus, they have $143,860 "too much" money to qualify for Medicaid ($300,000 – $154,140 – $2,000).
- **Income.** Once Isabelle is eligible for Medicaid, Mark is entitled to have income of *at least* $2,555 per month. Since his Social Security

and pension total only $1,600 per month, he will be allowed to keep $955 of his wife's income each month; the rest of Isabelle's income will have to be paid to the nursing home (less a small monthly "personal needs allowance" of $30-100 and occasional payments for certain medical expenses not covered by Medicaid). The Medicaid program will pick up the difference between her income and the nursing home cost.

④ **Estate Recovery.** Getting Isabelle on Medicaid is not the end of the problem. Even if Isabelle qualifies, the state will want to be repaid every dollar it spent on her care, following her death. Thus, some consideration must be paid to avoiding this "estate recovery." Otherwise, if Mark predeceases Isabelle and the house passes into her name alone, the house may have to be sold to repay the state, leaving her children little or nothing.

④ **What to Do First.** Because Isabelle's mental condition may deteriorate to the point where she can no longer legally sign anything, it is a good idea immediately to take her name off all assets so that Mark is the sole owner. This does not change the CSRA calculation, but it will permit Mark to make purchases and gifts even after Isabelle becomes incapacitated.

④ **How to "Spend Down" the $143,860 "Excess Assets."**

- Purchase a Medicaid-friendly annuity payable to Mark. This can absorb 100% of the excess assets and hasten Medicaid eligibility, but it will result in the loss of the ability to shift Isabelle's income to Mark and incurs the risk that Mark may die before Isabelle, exposing the annuity payments to estate recovery. See *Chapter 12: Annuities*, above, for a full discussion of this option.
- Prepay funeral and burial expenses of both spouses: estimated cost: $12,000-$20,000
- Prepay burial expenses of other family members: estimated cost: $3,000-$50,000 or more

- Improve the house: estimated cost: $15,000 (new heater/AC, new roof, etc.)
- Buy a newer auto for Mark: estimated cost: $10,000-$20,000 plus trade-in of old car
- Buy additional personal property (big screen TV, computer, grand piano, etc.): estimated cost: $6,000

  TOTAL OF ABOVE SPENDDOWN: $46,000-$111,000 or more

- If money is still left over after above expenditures, make a gift using the half-a-loaf technique; see below for calculations

④ **Half-a-Loaf Gifting.** After making the above expenditures (assume the bottom figure of $46,000 was all they could reasonably spend), there is still $97,860 ($143,860 - $46,000) of excess assets, before Isabelle will qualify for Medicaid. They should consider "half-a-loaf" gifting.

④ **Here's the Formula for the Amount of the Gift:** Divide the total amount of excess assets ($97,860) by the total of the couple's net monthly expenses ($4,250) + the penalty divisor ($5,000), which gives us this:

$97,860 ÷ (4,250 + 5,000) = $97,860 ÷ 9,250 = 10.6

Multiply the above number of months' penalty (10.6) x the penalty divisor ($5,000) = $53,000. Thus, Mark should make a gift of $53,000 to the children and use the balance of their excess assets ($44,860) to purchase a Medicaid-friendly annuity (with Mark as the owner and annuitant) or lend to the children in exchange for a promissory note.

Mark should then immediately apply for Medicaid for Isabelle, whereupon he will be told that because of the gift, Isabelle is disqualified for 7 months (of course, he already expected that, but he had to apply in order to get the penalty period running).

The annuity/note payments will increase Mark's monthly income for that 7-month period, allowing him to cover the private cost of

Isabelle's nursing home residency, and at the end of the period, he will have just below the CSRA of $154,140.

Proof: 10.6 x $4,250 = $45,050. This represents the total amount Mark will need to cover the nursing home expenses for the penalty period. Since this is slightly more than the total amount of the annuity payments ($44,860), the children will pay this small amount out of the gift they received at the beginning of this process. Were the annuity payments to be slightly more than needed, the children could use the difference to purchase one or more non-countable items for Mark's use, such as clothing or an item for the house. Depending on how much the penalty period is in your state and how much it costs to get an annuity, it may turn out that he will be a little short in the final month.

At that point, he can reapply for Medicaid on behalf of his wife, and, the penalty period having expired, she will immediately qualify, and all her nursing home bills will be paid by Medicaid.

Thus, *these techniques will save the family at least $99,000 out of the original excess of $143,860 (combining the "spenddown" of $46,000 with the Half-a-Loaf Gifting savings of $53,000).* Not bad for a "crisis" situation, where no advance planning had been done! Compare that to not doing anything and simply spending down the "excess assets" on Isabelle's nursing home care, which would have left the family with $-0-!

④ **Estate Recovery Issues**

As mentioned above, qualifying Isabelle for Medicaid is only half the battle. We must also plan for eventual estate recovery upon her death.

If she is the first to die, then there can be no estate recovery while Mark is still living, since federal law prevents a state from attempting to recover against the assets of a surviving spouse. However, upon Mark's later death, some states may attempt to seek reimbursement from a portion of his estate, under the theory that part of his estate really belonged to Isabelle; this depends on how they define "estate" within their state statutes and regulations.

In this case, the big asset is their house. Let's take a look at some of their options.

- ④ **How to Protect the House.** Let's first look to see what would happen if Mark and Isabelle did nothing with the house and then some possible solutions.
- ④ **Isabelle Dies First.** If Isabelle dies first and the home is still titled in joint names, some states will be able to file a recovery claim against her 50% interest. Most states, however, only look to the probate estate of the Medicaid recipient, so in those states, no recovery would be possible. If Isabelle dies first and the home has already been titled in Mark's name, then most states would not be able to make a claim against Isabelle's former interest in the home. In any event, no claim may be filed while Mark is still living.
- ④ **Mark Dies First.** If Mark is the first to die and the home is still titled in joint names, the house will pass into Isabelle's sole name. Thus, it will be part of her probate estate and subject to estate recovery in all states after she dies. That can cause a loss of the entire value of the home, depending on how long Isabelle lives while on Medicaid. If instead the home is retitled into Mark's name alone, then he may be able to leave Isabelle only a percentage interest in the house, enough to satisfy the "elective share" either outright or in a trust under his will (see Chapter 15).
- ④ **Gift Joint Interest in House.** Once the house is in Mark's name alone, he may be able to add one or more children onto the deed, ensuring that each owner is a "joint tenant with right of survivorship." That form of ownership ensures that upon Mark's death, his interest will not form part of the elective share amount. (NOTE: Elective share calculations can get very complex, since each state figures the elective share differently and may have laws that ignore gifts by one spouse that reduce the elective share owed to the other spouse. This is definitely something your elder law attorney must figure out for you!) Assuming Isabelle is already on Medicaid, it is probably okay for Mark to make a gift of an interest in the

house to their children without affecting Isabelle's eligibility. As discussed above, Mark needs to be aware that once he adds children to the deed, they are coowners of the house with him, so he cannot sell it without their permission and if they are sued or divorced or go bankrupt, the child's interest in the house could be attached, possibly causing him to lose his ability to live in the home. Also, he needs to keep in mind that if he needs nursing home or other care within the next five years, the gift he made to his children by adding their names to the deed will create a penalty that will affect his own eligibility for Medicaid.

In some states, it is possible to have unequal joint tenancy interests. If such is the case, then a tiny percentage interest can be given away, such as 1%, causing a very small gift. This can be important if a gift by Mark does indeed affect the eligibility of Isabelle. In that case, it would be important to make the gift as small as possible. Then, when Isabelle applies for Medicaid, she will only be faced with a very small penalty. The family would certainly be willing to bear that cost, in exchange for protecting the entire value of the house by virtue of the joint ownership deed.

④ **Gift House, Retain Life Estate.** Changing the house to joint ownership with one or more children exposes the house to the risk of a child being sued or divorced or going bankrupt, which could force a sale of the house. To protect Mark's right to continue to live in the house as long as he is able, and to protect it against creditors of his children, he can deed just a "remainder interest" in the house to his children (or to an irrevocable trust). This may be a better way to defeat the elective share, should Mark die before his wife. Since this is still a gift, the issue of whether this will affect Isabelle's eligibility must still be answered, based on the state rules.

- ④ **Transfer House to Trust.** Mark can also transfer his entire interest in the house into an irrevocable trust. The advantage is that he can continue to control the house, and possibly even serve as his own trustee, yet protect it against creditors of his children. This may also be a good way to defeat the elective share, since after a period of time the general rule is that the property can no longer be counted as part of Mark's property for such purposes. He can retain a right to live in the house for his lifetime, by reserving that right in the trust document. That can actually be useful for income tax purposes, since it will cause the basis of the house to be re-adjusted to the value on Mark's date of death; that can save the children capital gains taxes when they go to sell the house after their father's death.

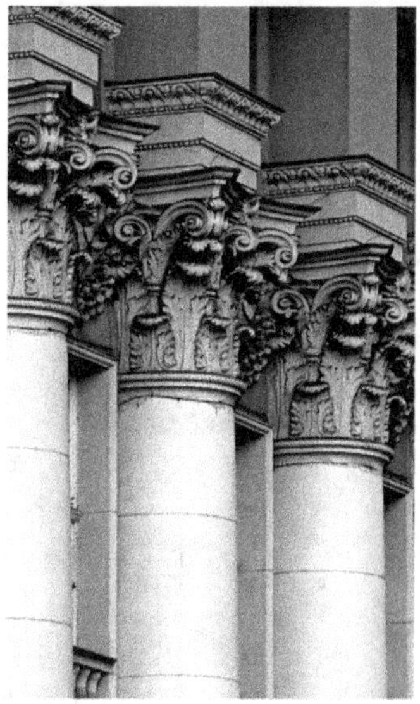

- ④ **Sell House, Move in with Child.** See discussion under Study #2, above.
- ④ **Plan for Mark.** Finally, no plan for a married couple is complete unless the possibility of *both* spouses needing longterm nursing home care is carefully considered and planned for. This study has focused only on obtaining Medicaid coverage for Isabelle; additional planning will also have to be done for Mark.

Study #4:

Married Couple with $950,000 in liquid assets, a home, and $9,000 monthly income. Two children, one disabled. ADVANCE PLANNING!

Sophie and Zelig have been married for 50 years. They have two children, Eric and Marsha. Marsha is disabled and currently lives in a group home.

Here are their combined assets:

Bank accounts and CDs	$100,000	W*
IRA	350,000	H
401(k)	150,000	W
Bonds	250,000	JT
Mutual funds and stocks	95,000	JT
Home	250,000	JT
2007 auto (Kelley Blue Book value)	5,000	JT

*Owned by husband (H), wife (W), or jointly (JT)

Their monthly income:

Social Security	$1,500	W
Social Security	1,500	H
Pension	3,000	H
Stock dividends	300	JT
Minimum distributions from IRAs	2,700	H&W

Their monthly expenses:

Health insurance premiums (Medicare Supp.)	$300
Miscellaneous personal (haircuts, toiletries, magazines, etc.)	200
Upkeep of house (average)	600
Groceries	400
Other	1,000

Let's go through this step-by-step.

- ④ **Total Assets.** The home and auto are excluded, so we don't count them for this purpose. Everything else is added up, regardless of whose name it is titled in: husband's, wife's or joint. Thus they have $945,000 in countable assets.
- ④ **Net Monthly Expenses.** The couple's typical monthly out-of-pocket expenses total $2,500.
- ④ **Wait...They're Millionaires! Should They Be Doing Medicaid Planning at All?** With over $1 million net worth and modest expenses, it would seem that they should not have to worry about long-term care expenses. However, should one or both of them need to enter a nursing home, their life savings would rapidly become depleted, because nursing homes in their area cost over $8,000 per month: That's $192,000 per year if both of them are in the nursing home! In addition, they are particularly concerned about preserving assets for their daughter, Marsha, since she will never be able to support herself.
- ④ **Medicaid Eligibility**
    - **Assets.** Since they don't know which one of them will need to enter the nursing home first, planning is difficult. In any event, the spouse at home ("Community Spouse") is limited to $154,140 (the CSRA), the nursing home spouse to $2,000, for a total of $156,140. Thus, they have an excess of $788,860 countable resources unless their state exempts their IRA/401(k) accounts, since they are already paying out minimum distributions.
    - **Income**. The Community Spouse is permitted to have income of at least $2,555 per month. If Zelig is the Community Spouse, his Social Security and pension exceed that amount, so Sophie's entire income will have to go to the nursing home. If Sophie is the Community Spouse, her income will also be higher than the

MMMNA of $2,555, because of the minimum required distributions from her $150,000 401(k) account. Even if they convert the 401(k) to an IRA and then use the IRA assets to purchase a Medicaid annuity within the IRA, the minimum distributions must still be made each year in order to avoid an income tax penalty.

- ④ **Estate Recovery.** Getting one of the couple on Medicaid is not the end of the problem: we must also consider estate recovery, i.e., once a person is on Medicaid, the state will want to be repaid every dollar it spent on the care of that person, following the person's death. In the case of Sophie and Zelig, the primary concern is the ultimate protection of their house.
- ④ **What to Do First.** Because this couple is not yet faced with the nursing home expense, they can implement some of the longer-term techniques discussed in this book.
- ④ **How to "Spend Down" the $788,860 "Excess Assets."** First, review the suggestions under Case #3, above.
- ④ In particular, they can easily **upgrade their 2007 auto with a new model,** thereby converting $40,000 or more into a noncountable asset.
- ④ **Half-a-loaf gifting is not advisable until one of them is ready to apply for nursing home care**, because you cannot get the penalty period started until you are otherwise eligible for Medicaid and actually apply.
- ④ Because of their timeline, **they should consider a gift of a large portion of their countable assets into an irrevocable trust** (Chapter 9). Because of the five-year lookback period that applies to this transfer, they should not apply for Medicaid until at least five years have passed from the date of the last transfer into the trust. But what if one of them needs to enter a nursing home before the end of the five-year period? To plan for this possibility, they must either (i) set aside an amount reasonably necessary to pay privately for nursing home care for the balance of the five-year period, or (ii) purchase long-term care insurance for this period.

If they cannot qualify for long-term care insurance, then they are in the position of having to guess how long it will be before one of them needs nursing home care and what the total cost will be. If they guess wrong and run out of money, then hopefully the trust will have been written with a "back door" to permit a distribution to their son, Eric; he could then use the distributed trust money to pay the nursing home until the five-year period expires and Medicaid coverage begins.

④ An alternative would be **a transfer of a portion of their countable assets into a Supplemental Needs Trust for their daughter, Marsha.** Such a transfer will not incur a Medicaid penalty. Another portion should go to their son, Eric, outright or in trust for him.

④ **Transferring their house to Marsha—or to a Supplemental Needs Trust for her**—incurs no gift penalty yet will prevent the state from coming after the house following the death of Zelig and Sophie under the estate recovery law. The parents can then sign a contract to pay a fair market rent to the trust, both guaranteeing them a place to live while further depleting their assets and making a transfer indirectly to Marsha in a way that is not considered a gift to her.

④ An alternative is to **transfer only a remainder interest in the house to a Supplemental Needs Trust for Marsha** (but be careful if your state has an expanded definition of "estate". The advantage of transferring only a remainder interest in the house is that the parents would at least be guaranteed the right to continue to live in their own home for the rest of their lives. The disadvantage would be the loss of the option to transfer rental income to Marsha's trust, which would further reduce their assets.

④ **IRA/401(k) Issues.** Unless their state exempts their IRA/401(k) accounts, because such a large portion of Sophie and Zelig's wealth is comprised of IRA and 401(k) money, they may be forced to liquidate most of those accounts. Unfortunately, doing so will incur a large income tax. Thus, if they can, they should try to withdraw part in one calendar year and the rest in another year; that will keep them in a lower tax bracket and ordinarily will save thousands in income taxes. It may also be possible for them to convert at least a portion of their IRA money into a fixed IRA annuity, making it non-countable for Medicaid purposes and also saving taxes by avoiding having to withdraw it all at once (see *IRAs and Converting to an Annuity*, Chapter 12). In order to do that with the 401(k), they will have to rollover the assets to an IRA first, as an intermediary step. Then they can convert the IRA assets to a Medicaid annuity inside of the new IRA.

Study #5:

Single woman with $300,000 in liquid assets, no home, and $1,600 monthly income. ADVANCE PLANNING!

Barbara is 77 years old. She has four children, only one of whom lives in her city. She lives on her own in an apartment.

Here are her assets:

Bank accounts and CDs	$100,000
IRA	50,000
401(k)	20,000
Saving bonds	30,000
Deferred variable annuity	100,000

Her monthly income:

Social Security	$1,050
Pension	250
Alimony	300

Her monthly expenses:

Rent	$750
Health insurance premiums (Medicare Supp.)	300
Home health aides	800
Groceries and meals out	500
Miscellaneous (haircuts, toiletries, etc.)	150

Let's go through this step-by-step.

- ④ **Total Assets.** Barbara does not own any excluded assets such as a home or auto (and the value of her used furniture and personal items is negligible). Thus, her total countable assets equal $300,000.
- ④ **Total Income.** Her income from all sources equals $1,600/month.
- ④ **Net Monthly Expenses.** Barbara's typical monthly out-of-pocket expenses total $2,500. Since that's more than her income, she's been dipping into her life savings to cover her living expenses.
- ④ **Concerns:** Barbara is still living on her own. Recently, however, she has had a series of strokes. Although she is now doing better, her children are concerned that if she gets worse and needs round-the-clock care, she will have to move to a nursing home. Knowing that the average cost of a nursing home in their mother's area is close to $7,500/month, they can see that this would rapidly deplete her assets. Accordingly, they want to find out if there is anything they can do to preserve and protect her assets for the future so that she will be in a position to qualify for Medicaid, should the time come when she needs nursing home care.
- ④ **First Thoughts.** Since we're not sure when—if ever—Barbara will need to move to a nursing home, the planning is more complicated. If she never enters a nursing home, she may well have enough money to support herself for the rest of her life, but if she needs nursing home care soon, she will undoubtedly exhaust her life savings. At that point she could apply for

Medicaid, but that leaves her children nothing, something that upsets Barbara very much.

Certain planning simply cannot be done in advance, such as half-aloaf gifting: in order to get the penalty period started, the applicant must be eligible for Medicaid "but for" any gifts made within the prior five years. So if a person is living independently, she cannot apply for Medicaid and therefore cannot get the penalty period started.

Transferring all of Barbara's assets into an irrevocable trust would protect those assets once five years has passed (that's the end of the "lookback period"), but such total divestment would be unacceptable to Barbara, a woman fiercely independent who is living on her own and who has always made her own decisions. After all, even though she could continue to receive trust income, she'd be giving up access to and control over the underlying assets in the trust (the principal), forever, when we're not even sure she'll ever need to move to a nursing home.

④ **Estate Recovery.** Since Barbara does not own a house, she is not concerned with estate recovery. After all, if her only assets other than her personal property are countable, and those assets must be reduced to less than $2,000 before she can qualify for Medicaid, then upon her death the most she can possibly have in her name would be $2,000 plus her personal property. In such a case, it's doubtful the state would even go after such a small estate.

④ **What to Do First.** If Barbara has not signed a Durable Power of Attorney that permits gifting and other Medicaid planning, she should sign one immediately. With her history of strokes, she could become incapacitated at any time, leaving her family unable to implement any Medicaid planning on her behalf without such a document.

Next, it's always best to consider **basic spenddown techniques**, before implementing any of the more complex techniques:

- consider purchasing an auto for the child who lives nearby to use to bring Barbara to the doctor, to family get-togethers, shopping, etc. The auto should be titled "JTWROS" with the daughter, to avoid possible estate recovery (in those states that do not go after joint property). This can easily protect $20,000 or more.
- pre-pay her funeral and burial expenses)
- pre-pay burial spaces for other family members, if desired
- sign a personal services contract if the child nearby is to provide more than occasional assistance to the mother
- upgrade her personal property (big screen TV, better audio system, etc.)

④ **What to Do with the "Excess Assets"**

- **Half-a-Loaf Gifting** is not advisable until Barbara is ready to apply for nursing home care, because she cannot get the penalty period started until she is otherwise eligible for Medicaid and actually applies. However, the entire family should thoroughly discuss and understand how it works so they are prepared to move fast should the need arise.
- An **irrevocable trust** while unacceptable to Barbara to hold *all* of her assets, will shelter whatever is transferred into it, starting five years from the date the assets are transferred. In addition, by retaining the right to all the trust income, Barbara will be able to continue her existing lifestyle. But Barbara is not in good health, and at age 77 she may need to enter a nursing home before the five-year lookback period expires.

Normally, it is advisable to wait until the lookback period has expired before applying for Medicaid, to avoid the imposition of a penalty. It works like this: if Barbara transfers $200,000 into an irrevocable trust and waits five years to apply for Medicaid, that money is ignored. But if she applies after, say, four years, there would be a penalty equal to the amount of the gift divided by her state's penalty divisor figure. Assume that the divisor for the state where Barbara lives is $5,000. That means there would be a penalty of $200,000 ÷ $5,000 = 40 months. And that 40-month penalty starts to run on the date she applies for Medicaid, giving no credit for the four years that already passed! But if she had waited another year, i.e., until the lookback period expired, she would have had *no* penalty. So by paying for 12 months—to reach the end of the lookback period—she avoids having to pay for 40 months.

But what if she needs to enter the nursing home after only one year? And how much of her remaining assets (after the above spenddown) *should* she put into the trust?

Let's take a look at how to analyze this:

- ④ Assume Barbara has about $270,000 to protect after doing the spenddown suggested above. Assume she transfers approximately one-third of these assets into an irrevocable income-only trust. So that means she transfers $90,000 into the trust and retains the balance, i.e., $180,000.

- ④ **Applying After Five Years.** If Barbara needs to enter the nursing home after five years, she can do the half-a-loaf method at that time. The $90,000 (plus its appreciation in value over the five-year period) is excluded in any event, so she is really able to protect *two-thirds* of her assets! One-third is excluded because it is outside the lookback period (the assets held in the trust), and another one-third is excluded via the half-a-loaf technique, which protects half of the two-thirds she never put into the trust. (If Barbara instead had transferred *50%* of her assets into the trust and she were able to wait at least five years to apply for Medicaid, then she could protect *three-fourths* of her assets: one-half is already protected because it was put into the trust more than five years ago, and the half-a-loaf plan protects half of the other half, i.e., three-fourths in total.)

- ④ **Applying Before Five Years.** If Barbara enters a nursing home before the end of the five-year lookback period, then what she should do depends on how close she is to the expiration of that period. If there are just a few months to go, she should pay the nursing home out of her own (non-trust) money for that time period, then do the half-a-loaf gift plan once she is past the five-year date. That will enable her to exclude the gift of the money into the trust from the half-a-loaf calculation (see above paragraph). If she does the half-a-loaf plan *before* the end of the five-year lookback period, then *the amount of the gift into the trust will have to be counted as part of the gifted amount,* significantly reducing the amount she can protect.

Example:

Barbara signs an irrevocable income-only trust, today, and transfers $90,000 into the trust, leaving her $180,000 outside the trust, titled in her own name. Two years from now her health deteriorates to the point where she needs to move into a nursing home. After working with her elder law attorney, she calculates the amount of a gift to her children as follows:

Half-a-Loaf Formula: Countable assets ÷ (net monthly expenses + state penalty divisor) = number of months penalty. Multiply that number by the state penalty divisor = amount to transfer. (Remember, the state penalty divisor in Barbara's state is $5,000.)

In Barbara's case, "countable assets" will have to include the $90,000 she transferred into the trust, because she's still within the five-year lookback period. Since she's now in the nursing home, we can accurately predict her monthly expenses, which are $7,500/ month. Subtract her monthly income from that number to get her net monthly expenses: $7,500 - $1,600 = $5,900. Thus, you take $270,000 ÷ ($5,900+ $5,000) = 24.8 months. 24.8 x $5 000 = $124,000. That's the amount of her gift under this formula.

However, *she already made a gift,* of the $90,000 she transferred into her trust two years ago. Thus, you need to subtract that from the target gift amount: $124,000 - $90,000 = $34,000. So all she needs to do is make an additional gift of $34,000 to her children and then purchase a Medicaid annuity with the balance of her assets. If she still has $180,000 outside the trust, then making a gift of $34,000 to her children leaves her with $146,000 with which to purchase a Medicaid annuity.

Proof:

Barbara needs $5,900/month for approximately 25 months, to cover the private pay costs of the nursing home during the penalty period. The $146,000 annuity should just about cover that: assuming *no interest* on the annuity (and there will always be *some* interest paid, or no one would buy annuities as investments), 25 equal payments will be $5,840, just $60/month short. If the annuity interest doesn't cover that shortfall, the kids will have to chip in, but that's a tiny amount. If even that is cumbersome, she can re-adjust the calculations so that she makes a slightly smaller gift, to ensure that she won't have to rely on her children's chipping in. After all, the nursing home's monthly cost may well increase in the next two years.

Conclusion: There's almost no downside to doing the trust. If Barbara needs nursing home care before five years pass, then she's in the same financial situation she'd be in had she done nothing, i.e., she is still able to protect 50% of her assets, using the half-a-loaf technique. (This assumes she does not fund the trust with *more* than 50% of her assets, to start with.) But, if she does not need nursing home care until *after* five years pass, then she can protect as much as *three-fourths* of her assets. So, she either breaks even or comes out ahead, using the trust. Of course, every situation is unique, and that's where you really need the input of an experienced elder law attorney to help you work through all these numbers, taking into consideration the health and financial condition of the elder facing a nursing home stay.

NOTE: Because the family was not sure how long it would be before Barbara needed nursing home care, they were forced to "hedge their bets" and not fund more than 50% of Barbara's assets into an irrevocable trust. Depending on how long it was before she needed to apply for Medicaid, they could protect either one-half or two-thirds of her assets. However, in the situation where you are fairly confident the parent won't need nursing home care for at least five years, the parent can certainly transfer more than 50% of his or her assets into an irrevocable trust. Indeed, if he or she transferred everything into the trust and lived off the income for at least five years, then the parent could protect 100% of the assets! If you guess wrong and need to pay for nursing home care before the five-year lookback period expires, you could always rely on the "back door" to access trust principal in an emergency.

Chapter 18

VETERANS PENSION: HOW IT WORKS

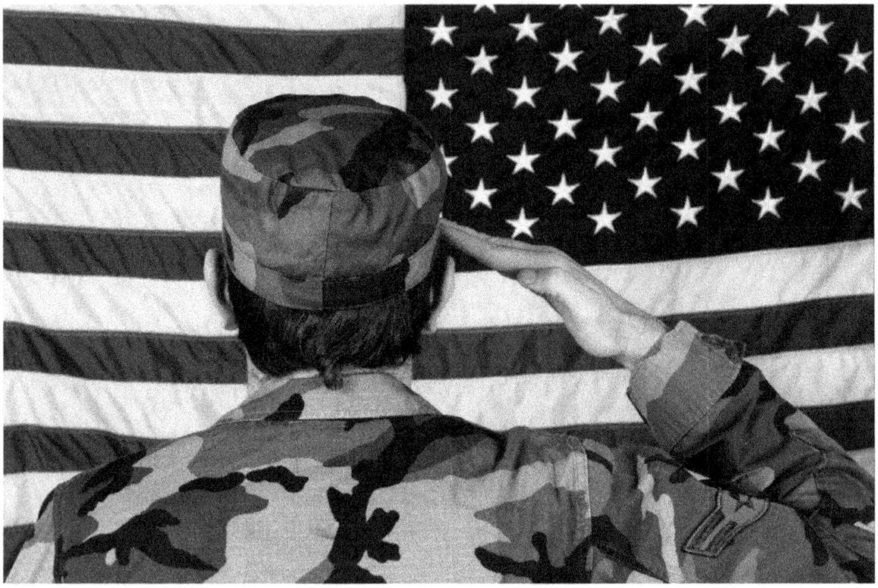

Introduction

There is a vastly under-utilized type of federal pension benefit that may be available to wartime veterans and surviving spouses who have in-home care or who live in nursing homes or assisted-living facilities. **approximately 11.5 million seniors—about 33% of all people in the U.S. over age 65—could qualify for a Veterans administration (Va) Pension or Death Pension by-meeting the tests outlined in this chapter.** That's how many war veterans or their surviving spouses there are in this country. Unfortunately, **fewer than 5% of those eligible for this benefit are actually receiving it.** A thorough understanding of these rules—and related planning opportunities—will help position you or your family member to qualify for these important federal benefits. This chapter and the next will enable you to do just that.

What is Pension?

Pension (for the veteran) and Death Pension (for the single surviving spouse of a deceased veteran) are supplemental income programs available to a veteran or to the surviving spouse. Payments are made to bring the veteran's (or spouse's) total income, including other retirement or Social Security income, to a level set by Congress. Charts showing the available amounts of income benefit are included below.

In order to receive the Pension benefit, a veteran household must meet the service requirements below, as well as meeting an income and an asset test and, in most cases, a medical needs test.

> **There is a sister benefit to Pension called Compensation. This is for veterans who are disabled because of injuries or illnesses incurred while on active duty. Compensation is generally the more desirable benefit for a number of reasons we will not go into here. A veteran household cannot receive Pension and Compensation at the same time. A decision must be made as to which benefit is better, and the veteran must choose only that benefit. If you may possibly qualify for**

Compensation, be sure to discuss this with your veterans' benefits counselor.

Eligibility Tests Service Requirement

The veteran has to have served on active duty at least 90 days with at least one of those days during a period of war (see table, below). There is no requirement that the veteran actually served in combat, only that the veteran was in the service *during* wartime and was discharged honorably.

Period of War	Beginning and Ending Dates
World War II	December 7, 1941 through December 31, 1946
Korean Conflict	June 27, 1950 through January 31, 1955
Vietnam Era	August 5, 1964 through May 7, 1975; for veterans who served "in country" before August 5, 1964, February 28, 1961 through May 7, 1975
Gulf War	August 2, 1990 through a date to be set by law or Presidential Proclamation

The Medical Needs Test

If the veteran is younger than age 65, he or she must be permanently and totally disabled to receive Pension. Medical evidence must be submitted with this type of application. If the veteran is age 65 or over, there is no disability requirement. For a single surviving spouse applying for a Death Pension benefit, there is no disability requirement, and neither must the deceased veteran have been disabled or at least age 65.

The VA will also provide additional income in the form of an "*aid and attendance*" allowance that is added to the basic Pension benefit if the veteran or the surviving spouse (i) is blind or nearly blind; (ii) is a patient in a nursing home because of mental or physical incapacity; or (iii) proves a need for the aid and attendance of another person to perform basic functions of everyday life, such as bathing, feeding, dressing, or going to the bathroom. Allowances are also granted if the beneficiary is "housebound" due to disability.

Unless the applicant is already a patient in a nursing home or blind or nearly blind, it will be necessary for the applicant to obtain a medical "rating" before the VA will award the additional aid and attendance or "housebound" benefit amounts. A medical "rating" is a determination by a Veterans Service Representative, after a review of the applicant's medical records,that the veteran or spouse applicant will either need aid and attendance or is "housebound" due to disability.

If the *non-veteran* spouse of a *living* veteran has a regular medical need for assistance or supervision, then, under certain conditions, a benefit (not an allowance) may be available for the veteran that otherwise would not be available.

Although, as indicated above, certain classes of veteran and spouse do not necessarily require a medical need to obtain Pension, in most cases a medical need for assistance or supervision due to disability *will* be crucial to getting the Pension benefit. A medical rating or a medical need for this disability care allows certain medical expenses and ancillary non-medical expenses to be annualized and subtracted from future annual income in order to meet the income test (see discussion, below). Most veteran households could not get the Pension benefit without this special provision allowing the deduction of annualized medical and non-medical-related expenses.

The high cost of medical and non-medical expenses associated with long-term care such as home care, assisted living, or nursing home care is usually the trigger that allows medical deductions to qualify a veteran household for Pension. That is why only 4.7% of all eligible individuals are actually receiving Pension. Other eligibles don't know about this special provision allowing them to meet the income test or they are currently not in need of long-term medical care.

The Income Test

Income is either "recurring" (e.g., Social Security or pensions) or "nonrecurring" (e.g., an inheritance or receipt of life insurance proceeds). Recurring income counts as income in the month received. Non-recurring income is really an asset, but it is divided by 12 and 1/12 is deemed received as income in each month for one year.

The household income of the veteran or the surviving spouse cannot exceed the Maximum Allowable Pension Rate (MAPR) for that category of application.

Countable income is all income attributable to the applicant, the applicant's spouse, and the applicant's dependent children. However, public assistance such as Supplemental Security Income is not considered income. As an example, using rates for 2024, a veteran and spouse with no medical rating cannot have a combined income of more than $1,806 a month or $21,674 a year from all sources. As another example, a single surviving spouse with an "aid and attendance" medical rating cannot make more than $1,477 a month or $17,743 a year from all sources.

If a potential applicant were to call a local regional office, the Veterans Service Representative (VSR) on the phone would typically ask about the amount of household income, the amount of assets, and the medical status. The VSR would check his or her table similar to the one below and if the household income exceeds the MAPR for that particular type of application category, the person calling the office would probably be told there is no benefit. *In many cases this is simply not true.* Keep in mind, however, some VSRs are aware of the special medical deduction and will give the correct advice in cases such as these.

Here's the key: If the veteran obtains a medical "rating," as discussed above, then *all* of the veteran's nursing home or assisted living costs can be counted as deductible medical expenses. The household income can then be reduced to meet the Pension income test. This allows households earning $2,000 to $6,000 or more a month to qualify even though their current non-adjusted income does not meet the income test (i.e., it exceeds the applicable MAPR).

Deductible Expenses: Once a medical "rating" is obtained, deductible expenses can also include the cost of paying a child for their services under a Personal Services Contract, as long as the child provides medical or nursing services for the parent. Examples of nursing services are assisting the parent with bathing, dressing, feeding him/herself, and other activities of daily living. The child or other caregiver does not have to be a licensed health professional. All reasonable fees paid to the caregiver for personal care of the parent and maintenance of the parent's immediate environment will be allowed. This includes such services as cooking and housecleaning for the parent.

If the parent is maintained in a home, assisted-living facility, or other institution, because they need to live in a protected environment, all unreimbursed fees paid for such custodial care ("room-and-board") and medical or nursing care are deductible expenses, as long as the parent receives a medical "rating" or a licensed physician certifies that the parent has a medical condition that makes such a level of care necessary.

Adult Day Care, Rest Homes, or Group Homes

If the veteran or spouse has a medical rating or is certified by a physician as needing the care provided by the facility, then the VA will allow a medical expense deduction for all reasonable fees paid to the facility as long as the facility provides some medical or nursing services for the disabled person. The services do not have to be furnished by a licensed health professional. If the veteran or spouse does not qualify under the above, then the VA will allow expenses paid to the facility "only to the extent that they represent payment for medical treatment furnished by a licensed health professional."

Home Care Costs. The special provision for annualizing and deducting non-medical costs associated with a rating also applies to home care costs. Home care costs can include the costs of assistance whether provided by professional aides, members of the family (other than the spouse), friends, or others hired independently to provide care in the home.

This special provision also applies to the non-veteran spouse receiving assisted living care or home care, but in this case there is no rating and no additional allowance. Another special rule, equivalent to a rating without an allowance, allows the spouse to deduct non-medical costs associated with assisted living or home care to be used for determining countable family income.

Example:

Suppose a veteran and spouse earn $4,000 a month and the veteran anticipates a medical need for "aid and attendance." They do not meet the 2024 income test of making less than $2,727 a month or $32,729 a year for this particular "aid and attendance" MAPR. Without the need for "aid and attendance," the MAPR for the income test is even more restrictive: $1,806 a month or $21,674 a year. They don't meet the income test for this alternative MAPR, either. However, VA will allow the household income to be reduced by any unreimbursed medical expenses that are incurred in the month of application or any expenses that are expected to recur regularly over the coming 12 months. A good example of a recurring expense is the cost of medical insurance such as Medicare Part B ($174.70—or more—a month for 2024).

In our example, the couple submits an application. VA will take all estimated sources of income over the next 12 months and add them together. Assume that the only source of income is the recurring $4,000 a month from Social Security and employer pensions. In this case, VA uses $48,000 as the starting point for the income test. Next, medical expenses are added up. Unreimbursed, ongoing prescription drug costs can also be applied toward medical expenses, but in this case, all prescription drugs are covered by insurance. The family reports Medicare Part B expenses of $350 a month (the amount both are paying). The veteran is also in an assisted living facility and is paying $3,500 a month ($42,000 a year) for the facility, which is also unreimbursed. Payment for assisted living is coming from savings and income. Recurring medical services provided by the assisted living facility can be deducted for the income test, and the assisted living facility reports that medical services from the assisted living personnel are $200 a month. Medical services include both services from a licensed health care practitioner and services provided for help with activities of daily living. The rest of the assisted living cost is for room and board and other ancillary services and cannot be deducted. As a result, allowable and deductible assisted living medical expenses for the income test only amount to $2,400 a year.

All medical expenses that are expected to recur every month over the next 12 months are added together and they total $6,600 ($350 + $200 = $550 x 12 = $6,600). Next, VA subtracts a medical expense deductible equal to 5% of the basic MAPR (without the allowance) which is $1,084. After the deduction, the allowable medical expense now totals $5,516. This amount is subtracted from the $48,000 anticipated, 12-month future income in order to arrive at a new income called "countable" income or IVAP (Income for VA Purposes). This new income figure will be used for the income test. The income test requires subtracting countable income from the maximum MAPR for this particular category of claim. If countable income exceeds the MAPR there is no benefit. If countable income is less than the MAPR, the difference between the two becomes the benefit. It is obvious this $5,516 medical expense will not bring the household countable income below the MAPR of $32,729 (or the alternative MAPR of $21,674 without aid and attendance) a year to pass the income test.

Benefit of Medical Rating. However, assuming the veteran gets a medical "rating," he can count his entire $42,000 assisted living costs towards determination of the household income test. Along with their other medical expenses they can now use $47,516 ($42,000 + $5,516) towards household medical expenses. Subtracting the allowable medical expenses amount from the household $48,000 income, the couple now has countable income of $484 which puts them well below the MAPR of $32,729 the ceiling for the income test with a rating and an allowance for "aid and attendance." Subtracting the countable income from MAPR ($32,729-$484) gives an award from VA of $32,245 per year or $2,686 a month in additional income. This is in addition to the income they are already making and will help cover the cost of the veteran's assisted living.

The Asset Test

As of October 18, 2018, the VA imposed a net worth limit. As of December 1, 2024, entitlement to VA pension requires that the applicant (and spouse, if any) not have more than $159,240 (figure re-adjusted annually) of net worth. For these purposes, "net worth" is the sum of countable assets AND annual countable income. This is much different than the Medicaid rules discussed above, which count assets and income separately and have separate limits for each category. Thus, for example, under these VA rules, if the countable assets of the claimant (and spouse, if any) are $145,000, and their annual countable income is $15,000, that total—$160,000—puts him over the VA limit, and VA pension will be denied (or discontinued if he had previously been receiving VA pension payments).

The value of mortgages and debt on included property is subtracted, *except* for any mortgage on the personal residence. Thus, the applicant would typically want to pay down and/or eliminate any mortgage on their primary residence, as a quick way of reducing their countable assets, if that is necessary to meet the above limitation.

To reduce assets, the veteran applicant can simply spend down part of his assets on himself, his spouse, child or relative (if the relative is living with the veteran, spouse, or child). Whatever is purchased must be for fair market value. Thus, the veteran applicant can purchase goods and/or services for any of the listed parties without it being considered a gift possibly causing a penalty period (see below regarding that topic).

Placing assets in a trust will not reduce assets assuming the veteran/ transferor still has access to those assets. If not, it may be treated as a gift, causing a penalty (see below).

It is important to remember that a claimant's reasonably predictable projected unreimbursed medical expenses can be deducted from income when calculating their net worth. Therefore, for many claimants who are paying in-home care or facility expenses for themselves or a dependent, the income component of net worth will be zero, and this issue will not be a concern.

Exempt Assets

The following assets are excluded from an applicant's countable assets when applying for VA pension:

Primary Residence. The value of a claimant's primary residence (single-family unit), including the residential lot area, in which the claimant has an ownership interest. VA recognizes one primary residence per claimant. If the residence is sold after pension entitlement is established, any net proceeds from the sale are exempt to the extent the proceeds are used to purchase another residence within the same calendar year as the year in which the sale occurred. The home continues to be exempt even if the claimant moves into a nursing home, other type care facility, or the home of a family member for health care or custodial care.

Residential lot area. The lot on which a residence sits that does not exceed two acres, unless the additional acreage is not marketable.

Personal effects. The value of personal effects suitable to and consistent with a reasonable mode of life, such as appliances and family transportation vehicles.

Other Exclusions: There are a small number of additional statutory exclusions from income and assets, listed in the Regulations, including, e.g., income tax refunds, food stamps, home energy assistance, etc.

Gifts

For the first time, the VA is penalizing gifts made to qualify for VA Pension, in a manner similar to that used for Medicaid qualification. There are a number of differences, however, discussed below.

"Covered Assets": First of all, the penalty only applies to gifts of assets that—had they not been given away—would have caused the claimant to exceed the asset limit discussed above. Such asset is called a "covered asset." Thus, for example, if a veteran claimant has assets that total $160,000 with zero income, and makes a gift of $50,000, only the amount that exceeds the asset limit for the year in question (currently $159,240) will be penalized, i.e., $760 ($160,000 - $159,240). Another way of looking at it is that the veteran only really needed to reduce his assets by $760 in order to meet the asset test, so any gifts that further reduced his assets would not have affected his ability to qualify for VA pension, and so they are ignored.

Example:

> A veteran with a net worth of $100,000 and zero income gives $90,000 to charity one year before she claims VA pension, leaving her $10,000 in a checking account. Because the gift of the $90,000 did not affect her VA pension eligibility (she would have qualified even if she had not made the gift), no penalty period is assessed.

Lookback Period: This means the 36-month period immediately preceding the date on which VA receives either an original pension claim or a new pension claim after a period of non-entitlement. Only gifts of covered assets that are transferred or gifted during this three-year period result in the imposition of a penalty.

Calculating the Penalty Period. If a transfer within the lookback period includes a covered asset, to figure out the length of the penalty, find the pension rate for a veteran in need of aid and attendance with one dependent that is in effect as of the date of the pension claim, divide by 12, and round down to the nearest whole dollar. Until December 1, 2025, that figure is

$33,548 ÷ 12 = $2,795.67. So a gift of $50,000 of covered assets would cause a penalty period of 17.88 months ($50,000 ÷ $2,795.67= 17.88).

The penalty period begins on the first day of the month that follows the date of the transfer. However, if there was more than one transfer, you must add up the value of all gifts of covered assets made within the lookback period, and the penalty period will begin on the first day of the month that follows the date of the last such transfer. Finally, if a penalty period is in force, the applicant will not be able to receive pension payments until the penalty period terminates. (However, in no event can the penalty period exceed 5 years, regardless of the amount transferred.)

NOTE: This is quite different from the Medicaid rules discussed earlier. Medicaid penalties do not start running until the date you actually apply for Medicaid, but under the VA rules the penalty period starts running even if you don't apply for VA pension until many months later.

Return of Assets. If the VA receives evidence showing that some or all covered assets were returned to the claimant before the date of claim or within 60 days after the date of VA's notice to the claimant of VA's decision concerning the penalty period, the VA will recalculate or eliminate the penalty period. For this exception to apply, the VA must receive the evidence no later than 90 days after the date of the VA's notice to the claimant of its decision concerning the penalty period.

Effective Date. Because these rules became effective on October 18, 2018, any asset transferred for less than fair market value before such date will not cause the imposition of a penalty period, regardless of the amount transferred.

Medicaid Planning. **It is also extremely important that if assets will be (or already have been) moved or otherwise rearranged, you should consult an elder law attorney with experience in Medicaid planning. It is very likely that the veteran or spouse may end up in a nursing home or end up paying more for care than the current income and veterans benefit combined. Nursing homes are very expensive, and the individual's income plus the veterans benefit rarely pay for the cost of**

a nursing home. This means the individual may have to rely on Medicaid to cover the deficit. Assets reallocated to qualify for VA benefits could create penalties for Medicaid eligibility, so it is vital also to plan for the possibility of needing Medicaid when doing your VA benefits planning.

How is Pension Calculated?

In general, you start by finding the correct Maximum Allowable Pension Rate (MAPR) for your situation. Then, you adjust it by subtracting all income, reduced by your unreimbursed medical expenses (the amount of which must itself be reduced by a "medical deduction" amount). The next sections will explain exactly how this is done.

Establishing the Maximum Allowable Pension Rate (MAPR)

Pension offers nine different maximum benefit amounts based on whether the award is for a veteran with a spouse or dependent child, a single veteran, or the single surviving spouse of a deceased veteran. For each of these three categories of benefits there are three levels of MAPR income depending on whether there is no rating, there is a rating for "housebound," or there is a rating for "aid and attendance." There are also rates associated with additional dependent children. Typically, an older veteran household will have dependent children if they have one or more totally disabled or cognitively impaired adult children living in the home. There may also be young, dependent children if the older veteran is married to a much younger spouse. In any event, if the household has such a situation, the additional dependent child rates are listed in the Table, below.

The calculation of each of these different categories of Pension income will allow for a benefit from zero dollars all the way up to the Maximum Allowable Pension Rate (MAPR) for that category. Here are the nine categories along with the maximum monthly Pension income for each category:

	Veteran and spouse with—
1.	no rating allowances—up to $1,851.33 per month
2.	housebound allowance—up to $2,165.17 per month
3.	aid and attendance allowance—up to $2,795.67 per month
	Single veteran with—
4.	no rating allowance—up to $1,413.75 per month
5.	housebound allowance—up to $1,727.66 per month
6.	aid and attendance allowance—up to $2,358.33 per month
	Surviving single spouse of a veteran with-
7.	no rating allowance—up to $948.33 per month
8.	housebound allowance—up to $1,159 per month
9.	aid and attendance allowance—up to $1,515.58 per month

Pension and Medicaid. Note that the "aid and attendance allowance" or "housebound allowance" portion of a Pension payment does not count as "income" for Medicaid purposes. This could be important should the veteran or spouse ever need to apply for Medicaid. Also note that while a VA pension recipient is not required to apply for Medicaid, a Medicaid applicant must apply for all benefits to which he or she may be entitled before Medicaid payments will be made to reimburse a facility. So a Medicaid applicant must determine if he or she may be entitled to VA Pension and if so, is required to apply for it.

$90 Pension Limit for Certain Nursing Home Patients. If a Pension or Death Pension recipient, *with no spouse or child*, is a patient in a nursing home and has qualified for Medicaid coverage, then the Pension or Death Pension amount cannot exceed $90 per month, after the end of the third full calendar month following the month of admission to a VA-run (VHA) nursing home or starting with eligibility for Medicaid in a private nursing home (after the month of admission). Veterans residing in state-run veterans homes are exempt from this $90-per-month limit. Such $90/month payment is not considered income and does not have to be paid to the nursing home, and it is paid in addition to the personal needs allowance.

Veteran's Spouse Eligibility. In order for the surviving spouse of an eligible veteran to qualify for Death Pension, the spouse not only must have been married to the veteran at the time of the veteran's death (they did not need to be living together), but the spouse cannot have ever remarried, unless the surviving spouse remarried and got divorced before November 1, 1990.

Doing the Calculation

Annualized future household income is totaled and annualized future medical expenses are added up and adjusted with a deductible that equals 5% of the basic MAPR. The adjusted medical expenses are then subtracted from the MAPR to create a new income called "countable income" or also known as IVAP (Income for Veterans Affairs Purposes). A negative IVAP is considered to be zero income. If the IVAP is less than the MAPR for a given application category, then it is subtracted from the MAPR and the difference becomes the annual benefit award for the veteran household. Benefits are paid monthly and therefore the award is divided by 12 and rounded down.

Examples

Here are some examples of calculating the Pension award based on three different application categories:

Example 1:

Single Surviving Spouse of a Deceased Qualifying Veteran. Surviving spouse is receiving paid home care with aid and attendance allowance. Her annual income is $11,000. Her unreimbursed medical expenses ($12,719) include prescription drugs, Medicare premiums, Medicare supplement premiums, and 12 months of prospective home health aide monthly costs.

Assume she meets the asset test.

Total 12-month future income from all sources	$11,000

Less 12 months future unreimbursed medical expenses reduced by 5% of MAPR [5% of MAPR ($11,102) = $555]	($12,164)
= Total countable income or IVAP	-$1,164
Single Death Pension MAPR with aid and attendance allowance	$17,743
Less countable income or IVAP (if negative, enter -0-)	($0)
= Yearly Pension award	$17,743
Monthly Pension award (yearly divided by 12)	$1,481

Example 2:

Veteran Couple with Veteran Paying the Medical Costs. Veteran is in assisted living with aid and attendance allowance; his spouse is living at home. Their annual family income is $48,000. Their unreimbursed medical expenses ($39,497) include prescription drugs, Medicare premiums, Medicare supplement premiums, and 12 months of prospective assisted living monthly costs. Assume the couple meets the asset test.

Total 12-month future income from all sources	$48,000
Less 12 months future unreimbursed medical expenses reduced by 5% of MAPR [5% of MAPR ($21,673) = $1,084]	($38,413) =
Total countable income or IVAP	$9,587
Couple's Pension MAPR with aid and attendance allowance	$32,729
Less countable income or IVAP	($9,587)
= Yearly Pension award	$23,142
Monthly Pension award (yearly divided by 12)	$1,929

Example 3:

Veteran Couple with Non-Veteran Spouse Paying the Medical Costs. Non-veteran spouse is receiving paid home care. Under VA rules she does not qualify for a rating but she does meet the special medical needs test. Annual family income is $32,000. Unreimbursed medical expenses ($32,034) include prescription drugs, Medicare premiums, Medicare supplement premiums, and 12 months of prospective home health aide monthly costs.

Assume they meet the asset test.

Total 12-month future income from all sources	$32,000
Less 12 months future unreimbursed medical expenses reduced by 5% of MAPR [5% of MAPR ($21,673) = $1,084]	($30,916)
= Total countable income or IVAP	$1,084
Couple's Pension MAPR *(no allowances available for these types of claims)*	$21,673
Less countable income or IVAP	($1,084)
= Yearly Pension award	$20,589
Monthly Pension award (yearly divided by 12)	$1,716

Chapter 19

VETERANS PENSION: PLANNING TECHNIQUES

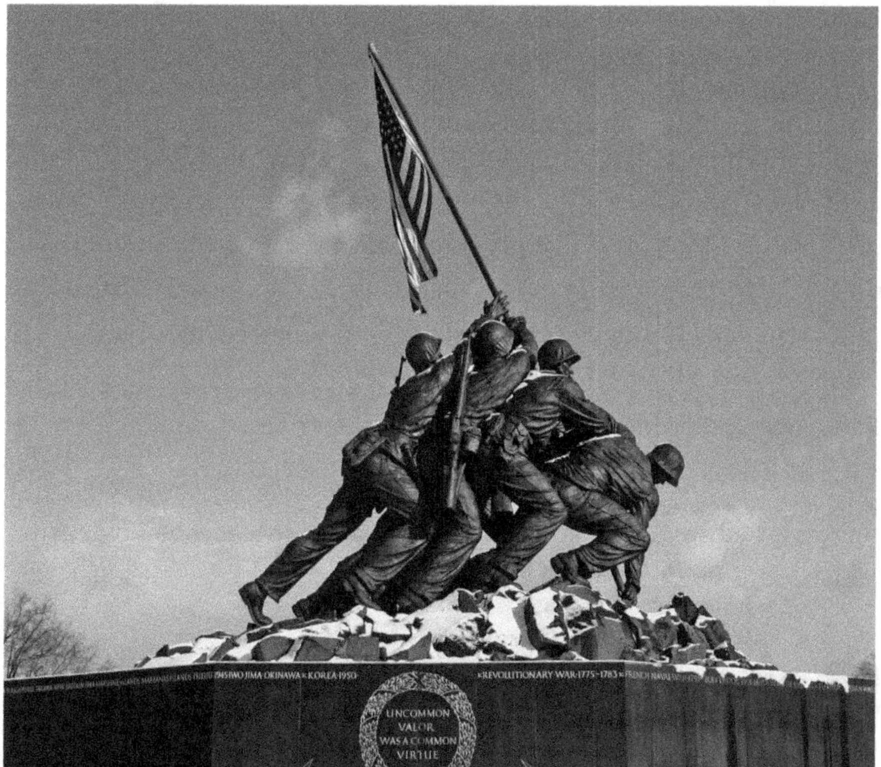

Assets Must Be Completely Divested Including No Life Estates

Any assets that are not exempt must be completely divested or they will be counted toward the determination of net worth. The VA regulations governing transfer of assets provide that a gift of property to someone other than a relative residing in the transferor's household will not be recognized as reducing the value of the transferor's estate unless it is clear that the transferor has relinquished *all* rights of ownership, including the right of control of the property. This means not only removal of ownership but also any interest or control over the asset, such as a life estate. This would also include trusts that allow for having access to the funds in the event of long-term care or other catastrophic needs or trusts that provide an income because this would also be considered having an interest in the gifted asset. A VA General Counsel opinion held that even an irrevocable self-settled supplementary needs trust is a countable asset for VA purposes. (Note that the veteran may safely serve as a trustee of a trust in which the veteran has no other interest, without that causing the trust to be a countable asset.)

Assets are also disregarded as a gift if they are given to someone residing in the household.

Exempt Assets

Since a personal residence, automobiles used for transportation, personal property that is not an investment, and up to two acres of the land on which the personal residence sits are exempt from the net worth determination, a good planning technique is to convert countable assets to one or more of these exempt assets. Thus, a veteran who is renting his living space may consider purchasing a condo or house and residing in it for some period of time before applying for VA pension. Another idea is to upgrade personal possessions such as a large-screen TV, better clothes for the whole family, or a new sprinkler system for the house, as well as paying for vacations for the veteran and other family members.

NOTE: A personal residence occupying land or sitting on a farm owned by the veteran or in the same building as a business is only exempt to the extent of the personal residence itself and the land on which it sits (up to a maximum of two acres). The balance of the property is considered part of the applicant's net worth for purposes of the asset test.

Converting Assets to Cash Should Not Result in Substantial Sacrifice

According to VA Manual M21-1MR,

> One factor to consider in making a net worth determination is whether or not the property can readily be converted into cash at no substantial sacrifice. This means that a claim should not be denied for excessive net worth if the claimant cannot convert assets into significant cash assets because of temporary market conditions or other reasons.
>
> However, if a piece of property can be converted into significant cash assets, it is immaterial that the property was worth more in the past or might be worth more in the future. The sole question to consider is how much money the claimant would receive if the property were sold at this time.

In essence, a claim cannot be denied if an asset that would count towards net worth cannot be converted into cash "without substantial sacrifice." This might include the effects of temporary market conditions or "other reasons." It is these other reasons that may allow planning opportunities for reallocating assets that do not rely on gifting those assets.

Planning Opportunities for Reallocating Assets to Qualify for Pension

Transfers at Least 36 Months Prior to Application

A transfer at least 36 months prior to application may be used to do legitimate estate planning, by transferring some assets into an irrevocable trust for the benefit of other family members. In order to ensure that the trust assets are not countable as part of the transferor veteran's assets for purposes of VA pension eligibility, the transferor cannot retain any interest in the trust.

It would also be possible for the veteran to purchase an immediate annuity, retaining monthly payments. While the annual income (payments) would be counted as part of the veteran's net worth for VA purposes, the lump sum that was paid to the annuity company will escape being so counted, once the three-year lookback period has passed.

Planning could be done with assets that would normally be gifted to the children when there is no pressing need to do so. The promise of a substantial benefit in the future could provide the incentive for transferring these assets now, to get the lookback period running as soon as possible. Planning for future veterans benefits would also lead to other estate planning such as wills, trusts, powers of attorney, appropriate tax strategies, and so forth. Of course, it is important for you to evaluate your possible future need for the gifted assets, because once they are given to your children, your children may or may not use—or even have—those assets to take care of you should the need arise at some point down the road!

Converting Assets into an Income Annuity

This strategy works by converting excess assets into income and still meeting the income test. If after application of deductible medical expenses the corrected income or IVAP is negative, the income can be brought up to a zero amount without affecting the Pension benefit. A single premium immediate income annuity may be purchased with part of the disqualifying assets to produce a guaranteed income over a certain period of years. This guaranteed income is designed to bring the IVAP up to a zero amount. If there is a concern about a future need for Medicaid eligibility, then the annuity might be structured to meet Medicaid rules. There may be reasons why the annuity could be structured differently even if Medicaid eligibility is not anticipated.

Example:

Going back to Example 1 in the previous chapter, note that after subtracting 12 months' future expected medical expenses from gross income, there was a negative amount of income, i.e., $1,164. When the Pension benefit was calculated, the amount below zero was ignored, so in effect, the applicant could have an additional $1,164 of income without affecting her Pension benefit. Accordingly, the applicant should be able to purchase a single premium immediate annuity that will pay her $97/month ($1,164/year). For a 75-year-old female, for example, this would cost around $12,500 for an immediate annuity with a guaranteed payout for at least 10 years (less than her life expectancy). Since this is a small amount and might be difficult to purchase from a commercial company, an alternative might be a private annuity or promissory note, if available in your state. It would have the same result of protecting additional assets without increasing countable income. Bottom line: More assets are sheltered, and additional income is generated to cover living expenses, without reducing the Pension payments.

Half-a-Loaf Gifting

Since the VA penalty period starts from the first of the month after the month in which the last gift is made (within the three years prior to the date of application), it would be possible to utilize the old "half-a-loaf" planning techniques that used to be common in Medicaid planning (see *Half-a-Loaf* discussion). However, because the amount of pension vs the amount of necessary living expenses may not be nearly as equal as with Medicaid (where the nursing home expense is reasonably equal to the Medicaid divisor), some careful calculations will be necessary to arrive at the correct amount to transfer.

For example, if a veteran applicant has $50,000 in excess assets, and would otherwise qualify for VA pension, a gift of that money will cause a penalty period of 18.3 months, as we've discussed above. If the veteran now must spend his own money on living expenses for that period of time— assume his living expenses equal the penalty divisor of $2,727 per month— at the end of the penalty period he will have spent $50,000 of his life's savings. Instead, if the veteran gifts $25,000 (resulting in a penalty period of 9.2 months) and keeps the other $25,000 to spend on living expenses, by the time the shorter penalty period has expired he will have spent only $25,000 out of his pocket. At that time, he can apply for VA pension, and since the penalty period has expired, he should be able to qualify immediately.

If his out-of-pocket expenses are lower than $2,727 per month, he can transfer more than half of his extra assets.

Going back to the half-a-loaf formula, let's assume he only needs $1,000/month to live. Applying that formula, we get:

[$50,000 ÷ ($1,000 + $2,727) = $50,000 ÷ $3,727 = 13.4 months penalty] X $2,727 = $36,541 to gift.

In other words, he can gift $36,541 to his children, for example, keeping $13,459 of the original $50,000 excess. The penalty period starts at the beginning of the following month, and he will face a penalty of 13.4 months. During those months he pays $1,000/month out of the extra money he did NOT gift. Thus, at the end of that period, he will be down to the asset limit to qualify for VA pension, and the penalty period will have expired, allowing him to qualify for VA pension immediately.

Result: He managed to transfer to family members the sum of $36,541 that he otherwise would have had to spend down before qualifying for VA pension.

For more information on applying for Veterans' Benefits, please visit www.veteransaidbenefit.org, where you can also order the 550-page book *How to Apply for Department of Veterans Affairs Benefits* (Senior Veterans Service

Alliance). This book contains a wealth of information that the VA does not volunteer to the public about how to receive a successful Pension award, and it also contains all the forms necessary to file a claim.

APPENDIX

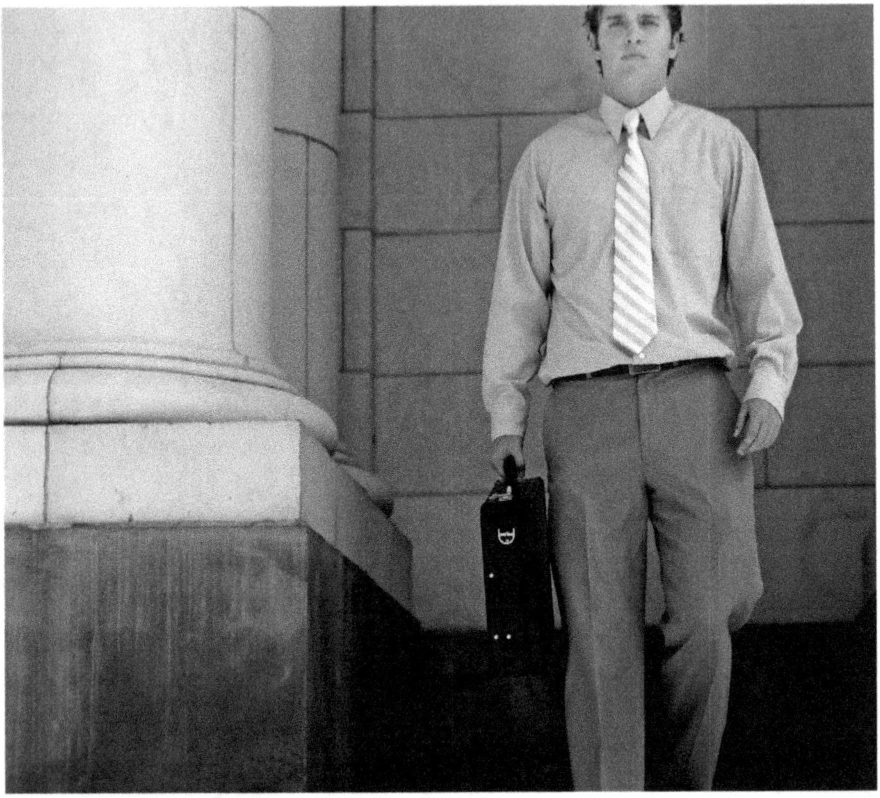

The Importance of a Durable Power of Attorney

As soon as possible, the family member who is the potential nursing home resident—whether that is your spouse, parent or other family member—should sign a comprehensive durable power of attorney. Without the power of attorney, should your family member become incompetent, there will be no one to sign documents or allow transfers and purchases for Medicaid planning purposes. Since the individual cannot sign, without the power of attorney you will be forced to hire a lawyer and seek appointment as the individual's guardian or conservator. Unfortunately, even with such appointment, you will need to have the approval of the judge in order to do any Medicaid planning-related transfers, and there is no guarantee you will get that approval. Some states actually have statutes that specifically authorize such transfers, but most do not. Since the primary purpose of the guardian/conservator is to protect the "ward" (i.e., the person who is under guardianship/conservatorship), the judge may be reluctant to permit transfers—even to family members—that will reduce or deplete the ward's assets.

Note that not just *any* durable power of attorney will do! The last thing you want to do is head out to your local office supply store for a $9.95 form, or purchase one (or obtain one for free) online. These basic forms will *not* contain the provisions you need to do Medicaid planning. For example, they rarely authorize gift giving and never mention Medicaid planning.

Even otherwise complete durable powers of attorney prepared by attorneys may not have the necessary Medicaid planning provisions. For example, they may omit the power to make gifts or may limit such gifts to the federal gift tax annual exclusion (currently $18,000 per person per year). Such a gift-giving limitation has its place in estate planning for the wealthy, but it can be severely limiting in a Medicaid planning context. Also, it should include the power to create and transfer the assets of the person signing it to a "special needs trust" for his or her own benefit, if doing so would allow that person access to any government benefits. Very important!

To be sure you have a power of attorney that will do what you need it to do, you really should hire an elder law attorney to prepare this document for you or your family member. Although the attorney's fee will be modest, it will certainly be more than the cost of the office supply form; however, it will be the best money you ever spent. With this properly prepared legal document, you will be able to make transfers to family members for Medicaid planning purposes without having to spend thousands of dollars going to court to be appointed a guardian or conservator, where you still risk having the judge turn down your request. Don't ignore the importance of this legal document!

Avoiding Non-attorney Assistance

A number of states have become plagued with non-attorney individuals or companies that aggressively market themselves as "Medicaid Estate Planners" or "Medicaid Asset Protection Specialists." By assisting the public with their Medicaid planning and applications, these non-attorneys may actually be engaging in the illegal "unauthorized practice of law." There have been several lawsuits shutting down some of the most egregious of these companies and individuals.

Too often the non-attorney individuals use inappropriate "Medicaid-friendly annuity" sales in order to quickly qualify their customers for Medicaid. Often there are more suitable options for the individual that are overlooked in favor of the annuity, which typically generates hefty commissions for the salesman while locking in the customer to an irrevocable and unchangeable investment or one with huge penalty fees if they decide to back out of it.

As you have certainly realized in reading this book, Medicaid planning is an extremely complicated area of the law. Do not trust your family's financial future to a non-lawyer who offers to quickly qualify your family member for Medicaid!

Same-Sex Marriage

On June 26, 2015, the United States Supreme Court ruled in *Obergefell v. Hodges* that state-level bans on same-sex marriage are unconstitutional. As a result, same-sex marriages are now legal and recognized in all 50 U.S. states, Washington, D.C., and the U.S. Territories. Thus, all the Medicaid laws—indeed, all federal marriage benefits of any kind—will now apply to same-sex married couples. A state cannot apply any different laws to a same-sex married couple: if a couple is legally married, then the spousal Medicaid rules apply to them, period.

However, it is important for same-sex couples to be aware of the potential downside of this change as well as the potential benefits. In many cases, a couple may be better off not getting married, once they focus on the potential disastrous financial consequences that may follow.

First, a clear benefit of being married: As discussed previously, a determination that a couple is married can in certain cases enable income to flow from the spouse in the nursing home to the Community Spouse, under the MMMNA rules. Since income only flows in one direction (i.e., from the nursing home spouse to the Community Spouse), getting married can only positively impact a same-sex couple seeking nursing home Medicaid eligibility under the income rules.

Unfortunately, frequently this benefit is outweighed by the consequences of the asset rules. That's because if the Community Spouse has assets of his or her own that total *more* than the CSRA, then being married can expose more of the couple's assets to a spenddown than with a similarly situated non-married couple.

EXAMPLE:

Barry, age 60, and John, age 65, decide to get married. Barry's net worth is $500,000 and John's is $100,000. Should John need nursing home care, not only will he have to reduce his own net worth to below $2,000 of countable assets, but Barry will have to spend down all of his assets in excess of the CSRA (currently $154,140). That's $345,860 of exposure! Had they simply lived together without getting married, then the full $500,000 of John's assets would be protected.

For a younger couple, this may be a remote issue, but for couples that are in their 60's and above, this is a very important issue that should be carefully considered in deciding whether or not to get married. Remember that a premarital/prenuptial agreement is completely ignored by the state when making an eligibility determination!

Of course, there are many other federal benefits that one member of a married couple would be entitled to that a single person would not be, such as spousal Social Security payments based on the work history of the other spouse, income tax treatment, immigration law issues, employee benefits, health insurance, etc.

Finally, see the section on getting divorced. The fact that more couples are getting divorced as a Medicaid planning option gives some indication that marriage is not always the best situation financially when one of a married couple is facing very expensive long-term care, and thus perhaps a same-sex couple should simply avoid getting married in the first place.

How to Find the Right Kind of Attorney

What you should not do: hire an attorney whose online webpage or other listing says "Divorce/Corporate Law/ Real Estate/Wills/Probate/Elder Law" (unless it is a firm with multiple attorneys with various specialties). There is simply no way one attorney can master all of these fields AND be competent in the specialized field of Medicaid planning.

What you should do: Locate an attorney who specializes in elder law, and particularly in Medicaid planning.

NAELA

A good place to start is at www.NAELA.org, which is the website for the National Association of Elder Law Attorneys (NAELA). Now just because some attorney paid a few hundred dollars and joined this voluntary organization does not guarantee any degree of competence in Medicaid planning. The truth is that NAELA is open to any licensed attorney, no matter how much or how little experience he or she has. However, it is also true that just about any attorney who specializes in elder law, and who makes it a point to keep up with this rapidly changing area of the law, will be a member of NAELA. At a minimum, it shows that the attorney has an interest in this area of the law and it's a good place to start your search.

At www.NAELA.org, after first clicking "Find a Lawyer," type in the zip code of the person for whom you are doing the planning. You can also limit your search to within 1, 5, 25, 50, or 100 miles from your indicated location, by clicking in the menu box to the right of the word "Distance." So if you live in Oregon, but you're concerned about your parents who reside in Massachusetts, then look for an attorney in Massachusetts, not Oregon. You want an attorney who is experienced with the laws, regulations, and local quirks of the state in which the person for whom you are doing the planning lives.

CELA Designation

There is one nationally recognized designation in the elder law field that actually means something. It is the "CELA" designation, which stands for "Certified Elder Law Attorney." There are currently slightly more than 500 CELAs in the U.S. Such designation is issued by the National Elder Law Foundation, and has the following requirements:

1. **Practice**—Attorney must have practiced law during the five years preceding his or her application and must still be practicing law.
2. **Integrity/Good Standing**—Attorney must be a member in good standing of the bars in all places in which he or she is licensed.
3. **Substantial Involvement**—Attorney must have spent an average of at least 16 hours per week practicing elder law during the three years preceding his or her application. In addition, he or she must have handled at least 60 elder law matters during those three years with a specified distribution among subjects as defined by the Foundation.

4. **Continuing Legal Education**—Attorney must have participated in at least 45 hours of continuing legal education in elder law during the preceding three years.
5. **Peer Review/Professional References**—Attorney must submit the names of five references from attorneys familiar with the attorney's competence and qualifications in elder law. These persons must themselves satisfy specified criteria.
6. **Examination**—Attorney must pass a full-day certification examination.
7. **Licensure**—Attorney must be licensed to practice law in at least one state or the District of Columbia.

Note, however, that NOT having the CELA designation is not a black mark against the attorney. This designation is relatively recent, many attorneys have a busy practice already and don't want the hassle of sitting for an exam to obtain a designation they really don't need, and others may not have the broad experience in different facets of elder law, yet have a deep experience in the narrow area of Medicaid planning.

While you cannot do a search on the NAELA website just for those attorneys with a CELA designation, it will show up on your search results page next to the names of all attorneys who have such a designation. However, you can also click the "Find an Attorney" link at the of the https://nelf.org/ website to search just for attorneys holding the CELA designation.

ACTEC

Another badge of expertise is membership in the American College of Trust and Estate Counsel (ACTEC). This "College" is not actually a school, but is a non-profit association composed of more than 2,400 of the most accomplished estate planning practitioners in the United States and Canada. A lawyer cannot apply for membership in the College; Fellows of the College are nominated by other Fellows in their geographic area and are elected by the membership at large. To qualify for membership, a lawyer must have at least 10 years of experience in the active practice of probate and trust law or estate planning.

Lawyers and law professors are elected to be Fellows by the other members, based on their outstanding professional reputation, exceptional skill, and substantial contributions to the field by lecturing, writing, teaching, and participating in bar activities. Historically, ACTEC attorneys have been considered the cream of the crop when it came to estate planning matters. However, recently some of them have extended their practice to include Medicaid planning as well.

Martindale-Hubbell®

Another measure of an attorney's expertise is his or her rating in Martindale-Hubbell®, the country's preeminent lawyer rating service. An AV® rating signifies a firm or attorney that has "achieved the highest levels of professional skill and integrity." The AV® rating is based on peer reviews by members of the Bar and Judiciary. That means that the lawyers and judges with whom the attorney has worked closely feel that the attorney is among the best in the business not only for his or her legal skills, but also for his or her honesty, integrity, and ethics. Attorney ratings can be found on the service's websites: www.martindale. com and www.lawyers.com.

State Certification

In recent years, many states have started to certify specialists in the law, such as bankruptcy, estate planning, litigation, divorce, etc. Some have also included the field of elder law as a specialty. Most states will piggy-back on the national CELA certification requirements, so once again that's a pretty good indication that the attorney is committed to this area of the law.

Secrets to Finding an Expert

Here's what I do, when looking to find an expert in any area of the law, when I do not have personal knowledge: go to the state bar association website and look for a list of current and past "CLE" ("continuing legal education") courses. Find one in the area of specialty you are interested in, and write down the names of all the attorneys who teach these courses. You can bet that the Bar

Association will not let someone without a good reputation as an expert in the field be an instructor to other attorneys! You will also be able to review the listed attorneys' experience, since the brochures for these courses typically list a short professional bio of the attorney instructors.

In addition to the state bar association courses, there are also a number of national firms that produce CLE seminars for profit. Once again, they will have done the legwork for you, by checking around with other attorneys in your state for names of experts to serve as instructors. Two of the biggest producers of these kinds of seminars are the National Business Institute (NBI) and the Professional Education Seminar Institute (PESI). Check out their websites at www. NBI-sems.com and www.PESI.com.

Who Is the Client?

Often family members other than or in addition to the potential Medicaid applicant will want to meet with the attorney. Although all family members generally want to save money if possible, some of the ways to do this may favor the younger generation at the expense of the older generation. Thus the elder law attorney must be careful to *identify who the client is.*

As a general rule, the person for whom the planning is being done, i.e., the potential Medicaid applicant and/or spouse, should be the client. This should be explained to all family members and also set out in a written fee agreement. The attorney will typically want to spend at least some time alone with the older generation to make sure that their wishes are fully understood and complied with. After all, *it is their money* that is the subject of the Medicaid planning, so they are the ones who should ultimately decide what they are comfortable doing or not doing.

For example, the attorney may come up with a recommendation that involves transferring 100% of the parent's money into an irrevocable trust. That may indeed be the best solution *on paper*, but it will leave the parent essentially impoverished and at the mercy of the trustee (who may or may not be the parent). The question must be asked: Is this the best option for the parent—or for the children? Sure, it offers the maximum protection of the parent's money, but at the expense of preventing the parent access to the parent's own funds! Thus, the children may try to persuade the parent to go along with this suggestion, since it is in the *children's* best interest, but the attorney must be careful that such planning is fully understood and agreed to by the parent.

Aggressive State Regulations

There is a trend among state legislatures to pass laws and/or issue regulations that are in clear violation of the federal Medicaid statutes. Apparently their approach is: "So sue me!" In other words, if an individual disagrees with the state's law or regulation, that individual can hire an attorney and sue the state, hoping to force a change or repeal of the illegal law or regulation. Of course, doing so forces the individual to spend thousands of dollars on legal fees, with no guarantee of a successful outcome (in some cases, the elderly client/plaintiff dies before the case has finished winding its way through the various levels of appeals within the legal system). The result is that the vast majority of residents of that state are required to give up legal rights and lose thousands of dollars in life savings, in order to comply with these illegal laws and regulations. The state knows this and is counting on this disparity in power to reduce the benefits it would otherwise have to pay out for its nursing home residents, thereby saving the state hundreds of thousands of dollars in Medicaid payments.

Note that even if a private attorney wanted to challenge the law or regulation for the benefit of all poor and elderly residents in his or her state, the attorney cannot do anything; in order to bring a legal action against the state in the hopes of changing the law or regulation, there must be an individual who is harmed as a result of the law or regulation. It takes a strong-willed and patient client—and one with deep pockets—who would be willing to be the plaintiff in a test case in the hopes of overturning the bad law or regulation.

Unfortunately, there is little the harmed individual resident can do under this system short of volunteering to be that test case.

2025 Figures

This book incorporates the 2025 federal figures for CSRA, MMMNA, etc. The MMMNA for the first half of 2025 was $2,555 (slightly higher in AK and HI).

This figure changes on July 1 of each year.

GLOSSARY

Activities of Daily Living (ADLs): Eating, toileting, transferring, bathing, dressing, and continence.

Agent: The person(s) who have legal authority to act on behalf of someone else, under a power of attorney document. *See* **Durable Power of Attorney**.

Aid and Attendance: A VA compensation or pension benefit awarded to a veteran (or spouse) who is determined to be in need of the regular aid and attendance of another person to perform basic functions of everyday life.

Annual Exclusion Gifts: Under federal gift tax laws, a certain amount of money or equivalent value assets may be gifted each year without requiring the filing of a federal gift tax return (Form 709). In 2024, this amount is $18,000 per gift recipient per year.

Asset: For purposes of the Medicaid transfer penalty rules, "assets" includes both income and resources. As used in this book, however, the term "assets" is limited to its more ordinary meaning, which would exclude a person's income.

Attorney-in-fact: *See* **Agent.**

Basis: The purchase price of an asset, increased by certain transaction costs (and, for real estate, improvements). Used in calculating capital gains taxes.

CELA ("Certified Elder Law Attorney"): A designation offered by the National Elder Law Foundation to attorneys who have met certain requirements indicating both substantial experience and expertise in elder law and who pass an all-day exam.

Community Spouse: The spouse who resides in the community, when one spouse of a married couple is in the nursing home. Also referred to as the "healthy spouse."

Countable Asset: An asset owned by the Medicaid applicant (or spouse) that is counted for purposes of determining Medicaid eligibility.

CSRA ("Community Spouse Resource Allowance"): The amount of countable resources permitted to be owned by the Community Spouse, in order for the Institutionalized Spouse to qualify for Medicaid. In 2024 this amount is $154,140.

Domicile: A person's permanent residence and the place to which a person intends to return should he or she leave such place temporarily. Thus, a person may have multiple residences (i.e., homes in several states or countries) but only one domicile.

DRA: The Deficit Reduction Act of 2005, a federal law that was signed on February 8, 2006. This law changed the calculation of transfer penalties, lookback period, treatment of annuities, etc.

Durable Power of Attorney: A legal document where one person (the "principal") authorizes another person (the "agent" or "attorney-in-fact") to act on behalf of—and in place of—the first person. It can be either "limited" (the agent only has the specific powers listed in the document) or "general" (broad powers to do whatever the principal could have done had the principal been competent). "Durable" means that the agent will continue to have the power to act on behalf of the principal even if the principal becomes incompetent.

Estate Recovery: The legal process of a state to seek reimbursement from the "estate" of a deceased Medicaid recipient for all the money it spent on that recipient's care, while that person was receiving Medicaid. "Estate" for these purposes is defined in various ways by different states.

Excess Shelter Allowance: If the "shelter" costs of a Community Spouse exceed the shelter standard (i.e., 30% of the MMMNA: currently $766.50), then the **MMMNA** may be increased, up to the **maximum MMMNA**, by the amount of such excess. "Shelter" costs are limited to the following: rent or mortgage (including both principal and interest payments), real estate taxes, homeowner's insurance, condo or coop maintenance fees, and utility costs (either a stateset standard amount or actual costs, depending on the state rule).

Excluded Asset: An asset owned by a Medicaid applicant (or spouse) that is not counted for purposes of determining Medicaid eligibility. Also known as a **non-countable asset or exempt asset.**

Exempt Asset: *See* **Excluded Asset.**

Fair Hearing: An administrative appeal within the state agency that makes the determinations of financial eligibility for Medicaid applicants. It is usually an informal proceeding, but bringing an elder law attorney is advisable.

Fraudulent Transfer: Also known as a fraudulent conveyance, such a transfer is one that is made by a debtor with actual intent to *hinder, delay, or defraud* any creditor of the debtor; or one that is made without receiving a reasonably equivalent value in exchange for the transfer, where the debtor was engaged or was about to engage in a transaction for which the remaining assets of the debtor were unreasonably small in relation to the transaction, or intended to incur, or believed or reasonably should have believed that he or she would incur, debts beyond his or her ability to pay as they became due. In short, someone making gifts in order to qualify for Medicaid could, in theory, have those gifts set aside and reversed by the state under this law, which is adopted in one form or another in all states. To date, this has not been invoked by states as a way to reverse Medicaid planning, but states may consider doing so at some point in the future.

Gifting Power: The specific authority in a **Durable Power of Attorney** to make gifts of your property to family members. This can be extremely valuable, allowing family members to do Medicaid planning for you even after you become incompetent. Unfortunately, most Powers of Attorney omit such authority.

Grantor: The person who creates and funds a trust.

HCBS ("Home and Community Based Services"): An optional state-provided Medicaid benefit to home-bound individuals who need nursing home level care.

Healthy Spouse: *See* **Community Spouse.**

Heirs: Those individuals entitled to receive a portion of a deceased person's probate estate upon such person's death, according to the laws of the person's state of domicile, if such person dies with no valid will.

Ill Spouse: *See* **Institutionalized Spouse.**

Institutionalized Spouse: The spouse who resides in the nursing home, when the other spouse of a married couple (i.e., the **Community Spouse**) is living in the community. Also referred to as the *nursing home spouse* or the *ill spouse.*

Inter Vivos Trust: A separate, stand-alone legal document that creates a trust.

It is effective immediately upon signing. *See* **Testamentary Trust.**

Intestate: Dying without a will. In such case, the law of the state where the deceased person had his or her last permanent residence (**domicile**) will set forth how such property must be distributed.

Intestate Succession: The procedure of distributing the probate assets of a person who died with no will. See **Intestate**.

Irrevocable Trust: A trust that may not be revoked or amended by the creator of the trust.

Joint Tenancy with Right of Survivorship ("JTWRoS"): Form of joint ownership of real estate where the interest of each owner passes automatically at death to the other (surviving) owner(s). *See* **Tenants in Common.**

Ladybird Deed supplemental needs: A deed that transfers the home to someone else, typically the transferor's children, while retaining the legal right to sell the house during the lifetime of the transferor, thereby avoiding probate. Not valid in all states.

Lien: A claim that is recorded in the registry of deeds office against a specific parcel of real estate, to ensure that the claim is satisfied before the real estate is sold. Title will not pass until the lien is released, so it is a way to guarantee that the property cannot be sold before satisfying the lien.

Life Estate: An interest in real estate that terminates upon the death of the owner of the interest. Until that time, the owner of the life estate has the right to the use and possession of the property and to the rents if it is rented out. *See* **Remainder Interest.**

Life Tenant: The owner of a life estate interest in a particular parcel of real estate. *See* **Remainder Interest.**

Living Trust: A trust that is created and operational during the lifetime of the creator. The term is usually used only to refer to a trust that is amendable and revocable by the creator. *See* **Testamentary Trust.**

Living Will: A legal document that states a person's wishes regarding termination of life support if the person has a terminal illness with no hope of recovery. Sometimes confused with a **living trust** because of the similar names, but they are completely different!

Lookback Period: The period of time prior to the date of a Medicaid application during which any gifts made by the person applying for Medicaid must be counted. The current lookback period in states that have adopted the DRA is 60 months.

MAPR (Maximum Allowable Pension Rate): The maximum allowable amount of income that a veteran (or spouse) may receive, in order to be eligible for the veterans Aid and Attendance pension benefit.

MMMNA ("The Minimum Monthly Maintenance Needs Allowance"): This is the minimum amount of income that a Community Spouse is entitled to have. If the Community Spouse has less than this amount, he or she is entitled to shift from the Institutionalized Spouse's income that amount of income necessary to increase the Community Spouse's income to the MMMNA. The

MMMNA is set by the federal government and changes annually. The MMMNA for the first half of 2025 was $2,555. This figure changes on July 1 of each year.

Maximum MMMNA: In certain cases, the **Community Spouse** may petition to increase his or her **MMMNA**, e.g., if the Community Spouse has high shelter related costs or other unusual expenses, such as very high personal medical costs. If such costs are approved, the MMMNA can be increased to as high as $3,854 (2025 figure).

NAELA ("The National Academy of Elder Law Attorneys"): A national organization with membership limited to attorneys. It is the pre-eminent such organization, holding national conferences that assist the ongoing education of its members. (www.NAELA.org)

Non-Countable Resource: *See* **Excluded Resource**

Penalty Divisor: The dollar number that is divided into the amount of a gift in order to determine the number of months of the **penalty period.** The divisor number varies from state to state and is typically updated annually to reflect the average monthly cost of a nursing home in the particular state (or region of the state, in some cases).

Penalty Period: The period of time during which an applicant for Medicaid coverage will be disqualified from such coverage, based on the amount of gifts made within the **lookback period.** *See* **Penalty Divisor.**

PoD ("Pay on Death") Account: A bank account that is immediately transferred into the name of one or more named beneficiaries upon the death of the original owner of the account. It is used to avoid having to probate the bank account, thereby allowing immediate access to the funds in the account following the account owner's death.

Pooled Trust: A state-chartered charitable organization specifically created to hold contributions of many disabled individuals, for the **supplemental needs**

of each disabled individual. Each contribution is maintained in a separate account for the lifetime of the individual.

Power of Appointment: A power to change the distribution of trust assets from that which is set forth in the trust document. Such power may be exercised during the power-holder's lifetime or only following the power-holder's death (a so-called "testamentary power of appointment"). The trust document itself will set forth the conditions of exercise, e.g., must be exercised in the power-holder's will, etc.

Principal: The term *principal* of a trust refers to the underlying assets (cash, stocks, bonds, real estate, etc.) titled in the name of the trust. Any interest, dividends, rent, etc., that are generated by these assets make up the trust *income.*

Probate Estate: The assets owned by an individual upon death that pass under the provisions of a will (or, if there is no will, by **intestate succession**). It includes all assets in the individual's sole name and excludes all assets that pass by right of survivorship (such as most jointly owned property) or beneficiary designation (such as life insurance, annuities, IRAs 401(k)s, POD, TOD, etc.) or that are held in the name of a trust.

Remainder Beneficiary: Also known as *remainderman.* The individual who succeeds to the interest in real estate after the death of a person who owned a **life estate** in such property; also the individual who succeeds to an interest in a trust after the death of a prior beneficiary.

Remainder Interest: The interest in real estate that comes into the possession of the remainder beneficiaries upon the death of the owner of a **life estate.**

Example:

Mr. Smith owns Smith Farm. He deeds the farm to his children, reserving a **life estate.** The children have no rights to possession of the farm until Mr. Smith's death. Upon his death, all of the children own the farm equally. Thus, during Mr. Smith's lifetime, the children are the **remainder beneficiaries** and own a **remainder interest** in the farm.

Resource: Any property (both real and personal) owned by a Medicaid applicant (or spouse), which is evaluated for purposes of determining Medicaid eligibility. Such resource may be **countable, unavailable, or excluded (exempt).**

Revocable Trust: A trust that may be revoked and amended at any time by the creator of the trust.

Self-Settled Trust: A trust funded with the assets of (and typically also created by) an individual for such individual's own benefit. *See* **Third-Party-Created Trust.**

Settlor: *See* **Grantor.**

Single: As used in this book, "single" means a person who was never married or who is divorced or widowed.

Special Needs Trust: A trust that is specifically created to distribute its assets for the benefit of a disabled individual in such a way that the trust will not disqualify the individual from receiving various government benefits. For these purposes, "special needs" are defined as those benefits and services that supplement but do not supplant, replace, or reduce otherwise available government benefits. Also known as a **Supplemental Needs Trust.**

Spend Down: The process of reducing the **countable assets** of a Medicaid applicant through various purchases and expenditures, so that the applicant will qualify for Medicaid coverage. The amount of excess assets is called the **spenddown** amount.

SSDI ("Social Security Disability Income"): A federal program that provides a minimal amount of income to individuals who are disabled as defined under the Social Security rules. Eligibility for these benefits is not based on the individual's income or assets.

SSI ("Supplemental Security Income"): A federal program that provides a minimal amount of income to individuals with very low assets and income. Many of the Medicaid asset and income rules are based on the SSI rules.

Supplemental Needs Trust: *See* **Special Needs Trust.**

Tangible Personal Property: Personal property that you can physically touch, such as furniture, a car, or jewelry. Thus, a stock or bond is not tangible personal property, because the paper it is printed on represents an ownership interest in something other than the actual piece of paper.

TEFRA Lien: A **lien** imposed on the residence of a Medicaid recipient during the recipient's lifetime to ensure that the house cannot be sold without first repaying the amount of Medicaid expenditures made by the state on behalf of the Medicaid recipient. This law was first enacted as part of the federal Tax Equity and Fiscal Responsibility Act ("TEFRA") of 1982. *See* **Lien.**

Tenants by the Entirety: A form of joint ownership of real estate where the only owners are a married couple. It offers some creditor protection to the spouses not available to non-spouses, in addition to the right of survivorship. It is not available in all states.

Tenants in Common: A form of joint ownership of real estate where, upon the death of each joint owner, such owner's percentage share of the property passes by the owner's will and not to the other joint owners. *See* **Joint**

Tenancy with Right of Survivorship.

Testamentary Trust: A trust created within the provisions of a will. Thus, it only becomes effective following the death of the creator of the will.

Third-Party-Created Trust: A trust created and funded by someone other than the beneficiary or his or her spouse.

TOD ("Transfer on Death") Account: TOD accounts are available for most types of "paper" assets, such as savings and checking accounts in banks and credit unions, certificates of deposit, stocks, bonds, and other securities. Such accounts are immediately transferred into the name of a named beneficiary upon the death of the original owner. They are used to avoid having to probate the account or certificate and immediately pass title to the beneficiary following the original owner's death.

Transfer Without Fair Consideration: A gift. For example, selling one's house to one's children for $1 is really a gift of the full value of the house, less $1. Such a transfer is without fair consideration, since the amount received by the seller was not the full value of the house.

Trust: A form of divided ownership: one person (the trustee) takes title to an asset for the benefit of another person (the beneficiary). It is essentially an agreement between the creator of the trust (known as the **grantor** or **settlor**) and the trustee, who oversees the trust property. The terms of the agreement are set forth in the trust document itself. A trust can be a free-standing, separate document (such as a **revocable trust** or **living trust** or **inter vivos trust**) or contained within the terms of a will (a **testamentary trust**).

Trustee: The individual or entity who manages and invests the trust assets and also determines the amount and frequency of distributions to the person or persons who benefit from such distributions (the beneficiaries of the trust). Many times family members serve as trustees for other family members, or a bank or trust company may be employed to do so.

Unavailable Resource: An asset that cannot be sold by the Medicaid applicant for legal reasons, e.g., an interest in an estate prior to distribution, an interest in ongoing litigation, etc.

ANNUITY (LIFE EXPECTANCY) TABLE

2021 Period Life Table, Office of the Chief Actuary, Social Security Administration

	Male	Female
Exact age	Life expectancy	Life expectancy
50	28.12	32.07
51	27.30	31.20
52	26.50	30.33
53	25.70	29.47
54	24.91	28.62
55	24.14	27.77
56	23.37	26.93
57	22.61	26.10
58	21.87	25.27
59	21.13	24.46
60	20.41	23.65
61	19.70	22.86
62	19.00	22.07
63	18.31	21.29
64	17.63	20.52
65	16.95	19.75
76	10.05	11.83
77	9.49	11.19
78	8.95	10.57
79	8.42	9.96
80	7.92	9.38
81	7.43	8.81
82	6.96	8.26
83	6.50	7.73
84	6.07	7.21
85	5.65	6.72
86	5.26	6.26
87	4.88	5.82
88	4.53	5.41
89	4.21	5.02
90	3.90	4.65
91	3.62	4.31

66	16.29	18.99
67	15.63	18.23
68	14.98	17.48
69	14.33	16.74
70	13.69	16.00
71	13.06	15.27
72	12.43	14.56
73	11.82	13.85
74	11.21	13.16
75	10.62	12.49

92	3.36	3.99
93	3.14	3.71
94	2.94	3.45
95	2.76	3.22
96	2.60	3.01
97	2.45	2.82
98	2.32	2.66
99	2.20	2.50
100	2.09	2.35

Source: https://www.ssa.gov/oact/STATS/table4c6.html

LIFE ESTATE TABLE (UNISEX)

Age	Life Estate	Remainder	Age	Life Estate	Remainder
50	0.84743	0.15257	76	0.50441	0.49559
51	0.83674	0.16126	77	0.48742	0.51258
52	0.82969	0.17031	78	0.47049	0.52951
53	0.82028	0.17972	79	0.45357	0.55243
54	0.81054	0.18946	80	0.43659	0.56341
55	0.80046	0.19954	81	0.41967	0.58033
56	0.79006	0.20994	82	0.40295	0.59705
57	0.77931	0.22069	83	0.38642	0.61358
58	0.76822	0.23178	84	0.36998	0.63002
59	0.75675	0.24325	85	0.35359	0.64641
60	0.74491	0.25509	86	0.33764	0.66236
61	0.73267	0.26733	87	0.32262	0.67738
62	0.72002	0.27998	88	0.30859	0.69141
63	0.70696	0.29304	89	0.29526	0.70474
64	0.69352	0.30648	90	0.28221	0.71779
65	0.6797	0.3203	91	0.26955	0.73045
66	0.66551	0.33449	92	0.25771	0.74229
67	0.65098	0.34902	93	0.24692	0.75308

68	0.6361	0.3639	94	0.23728	0.76272
69	0.62086	0.37914	95	0.22887	0.77113
70	0.60522	0.39478	96	0.22181	0.77819
71	0.58914	0.41086	97	0.21550	0.78450
72	0.57261	0.42739	98	0.21000	0.79000
73	0.55571	0.44429	99	0.20486	0.79514
74	0.53862	0.46138	100	0.19975	0.80025
75	0.52149	0.47851			

Source: https://www.irs.gov/retirement-plans/actuarial-tables

STATE NUMBERS

To find the latest Medicaid-related figures for your state, go to https://www.medicaidplanningassistance.org/state-specific-medicaid-eligibility/

As a general rule, these figures are updated annually each January, but a few states issue them a bit later in the year. As a result, it is important to verify them by checking with the State Medicaid Agency in your state before taking any action in reliance on these figures.

Here are the important numbers you will want to find, for your own state:

1. Individual Resource Allowance

Although the maximum amount of countable assets each Medicaid recipient in a nursing home is permitted to have in his or her name is normally limited to $2,000, some states allow a higher or lower amount.

2. Divestment Penalty Divisor

This figure is based on the average monthly cost of a nursing home in the state (or subdivision of the state, in some cases). This is the number used to calculate the penalty period that results from making a gift when no exception applies.

3. Monthly Maintenance Needs Allowance (MMMNA)

Find the minimum and maximum amount of income the Community Spouse is entitled to protect. If there is only one number, that means that the state permits the Community Spouse to protect the higher amount in all cases.

4. Shelter Standard/Standard Utility Allowance

Used in calculating if the Community Spouse has "shelter" expenses sufficiently high to permit an increased MMMNA, in those states with both a minimum and maximum MMMNA. In some states you need to add in the actual utility costs to arrive at your "shelter" costs; other states allow you to use the standard utility numbers. Finally, a few states allow you to choose which is more advantageous to you.

5. Community Spouse Resource Allowance (CSRA)

Lists the amount of "protected" assets allowed to the Community Spouse. If there is only one number, it means the state is a "100% state," and the Community Spouse can protect that full amount, but not more. If there are two numbers, it's a "50% state": the first number represents the minimum amount the Community Spouse is permitted to protect, even if 50% of the couple's total assets is less than that amount, and the second number is the most the Community Spouse can protect even if 50% of the total assets is more than that.

FEDERAL STATUTES

- ④ **42 U.S.C. § 1396**—Codification of Title XIX of the Social Security Act contains the Medicaid rules.
- ④ **42 U.S.C. § 1396p**—Liens, adjustments and recoveries, and transfers of assets. Here's where you'll find the rules governing gift penalty calculations, lookback periods, liens against the home, estate recovery after death, annuities, and trusts.
- ④ **42 U.S.C. § 1396r-5**—Treatment of income and resources for certain institutionalized spouses. Sets forth the rules governing spouses, where one applies for Medicaid: Attribution of income and assets, MMMNA, CSRA, etc.
- ④ **42 U.S.C. § 1381/1382**—The SSI program rules (also used for Medicaid eligibility in the majority of states)
- ④ **42 U.S.C. § 1382a**—Income; earned and unearned income defined; exclusions from income
- ④ **42 U.S.C. § 1382b**—Resources: exclusions, transfers, trusts
- ④ **42 U.S.C. § 1382c**—Definitions

Note that even though the Medicaid program is created by these federal statutes, the states are given leeway in interpreting many of these sections, resulting in uncertainty and discrepancies from state to state. If your state's own statutes, regulations or policies conflict with the federal law, an experienced elder law attorney will know whether to challenge the state in court and your likely chances of success. You should consider this option if the stakes in your personal situation are high enough.

RESOURCES

- Finding a good attorney:
    a) www.NAELA.org The main site of the National Academy of Elder-Law Attorneys. Here's where you can search for an elder law attorney by zip code, specialty, etc.
    b) www.specialneedsalliance.org Member attorneys are exceedingly experienced in drafting Special Needs Trusts and Supplemental Needs Trusts in order to protect a client's access to public benefits like Medicaid and Supplemental Security Income (SSI). Membership is based on demonstrated expertise and is by invitation only.
    c) www.lcplfa.org The Life Care Planning Law Firms Association is a national network of holistic law practices that offer legal services, care coordination and advocacy services to help elderly clients and their families navigate the long-term care maze. Life Care Planning Law Firms rely on an inter-disciplinary team that includes elder care co-ordinators as well as elder law attorneys, who work to identify present and potential future care needs, locate appropriate care, and ensure high-quality care. This approach relies less on crisis-oriented transactions and more on the development of ongoing relationships with families. In addition to traditional asset-focused elder law services such as estate planning, asset protection and public benefits qualification, a Life Care Planning Law Firm typically provides guidance for care coordination, family education and decision-making, nursing home advocacy, crisis intervention support and other services.
    d) https://www.longtermcarelink.net/ Here you can locate an elder law attorney who also is experienced in handling VA pension matters. In addition, the site is a comprehensive resource for

eldercare, senior services and care planning articles, books, and guides.

- Finding a good nursing home:
  a) https://www.medicare.gov/publications/12130nursing-home-checklist508.pdf A great checklist of what to look for when selecting a nursing home.
  b) https://www.medicare.gov/care-compare/?redirect=true&providerType=NursingHome Find detailed information about every Medicare and Medicaid-certified nursing home in the country. A great resource!
  c) https://www.medicare.gov/sites/default/files/2024-07/02174-your-guide-to-choosing-a-nursing-home.pdf Useful booklet on how to select a good nursing home.
  d) https://www.genworth.com/aging-and-you/finances/cost-of-care Useful online tool allows you to look up the average costs of care in different states in the U.S. Shows the costs of home health care, adult day health care, assisted living facilities, and nursing homes.

- www.elderlawanswers.com Information on elder law topics; resources; attorney lists; and a unique discussion forum where you can post questions and read others' answers. Also includes a search function to find an elder law attorney in your area.
- https://murphyberglund.com/medicaid-va-benefits/ Author's website with glossary of terms
- http://www.Medicaid.gov The main Medicaid page of the federal body that governs the Medicaid program, the Centers for Medicare and Medicaid Services ("CMS"). Here you can find detailed information on the Medicaid program, as well as links to relevant statutes, regulations, and agency letters.
- https://secure.ssa.gov/apps10/ Links to the various sections of the "POMS" (Social Security's *Program Operations Manual System*), which contains

regulations and statutory policy interpretations that govern the Medicaid program.

- https://www.va.gov/opa/publications/benefits_book/2023_Federal_Benefits_for_Veterans_Dependents_and_Survivors.pdf. Links you to *Federal Benefits for Veterans, Dependents, and Survivors (2023 edition)*, a helpful book published by the federal government detailing various veterans benefits, including Aid and Attendance. Now available as a free pdf download or read all the chapters online.
- https://www.benefits.gov/categories/ List of various benefits categories. Click "Healthcare and Medical Assistance" for information on Medicaid eligibility.
- www.MedicaidAnnuity.com Krause Financial Services. Headed up by Dale Krause, who is an attorney, this company specializes in Medicaid annuities. Dale is very active with the elder law bar across the country and is very knowledgeable about this area. Also includes Planning Tools (intake forms, quote forms, etc.), Agent Tools (agent-only forum, applications, etc.), the Krause Report (guide to using insurance products in Medicaid and VA planning), and State-specific Resources (state "numbers," annuity rules, etc.).

CHECKLIST OF MEDICAID PLANNING OPTIONS

This checklist is designed to serve as a "memory jogger" as you focus on the facts of your own situation, to prevent you from overlooking a helpful technique. Of course, as you have learned, not every technique applies in every state!

Single Clients

1. Convert Countable to Exempt (no penalty, no lookback)

    a) Medicaid Annuity

        i. purchase
        ii. convert retirement plan

    b) Promissory note
    c) Tangible Personal Property
    d) Auto: new purchase or upgrade
    e) Home: new purchase or upgrade
    f) Home improvements
    g) Life estate purchase in child's home
    h) Joint purchase of interest in child's home
    i) Joint purchase of house w child
    j) Funeral/burial funds and spaces
    k) Income-producing property
    l) Property used in trade or business
    m) Single premium life insurance policy
    n) Personal services contract

        iii. ongoing
        iv. lump sum in advance ("life care")

2. Gifting (causes penalty or must wait 5 years)

   a) Half-a-loaf
   b) Reverse half-a-loaf (where permitted)
   c) Irrevocable trust
   d) Gift to irrev trust, retain life estate
   e) Gift to children, then trust or bank account for parents
   f) House to child, retaining life estate
   g) Gifts + purchase of decreasing-term LTCI

3. No-Penalty Gifting

   a) Already exempt assets (other than the home)
   b) (d)(4)(A) trust (self-funded disability trust)
   c) (d)(4)C) trust (pooled trust)
   d) To blind or disabled child (outright)
   e) To trust for blind or disabled child
   f) To trust for disabled person under 65
   g) House

      i. to blind or disabled child
         - outright, or
         - in trust
      ii. to sibling w equity interest
      iii. to caretaker child

Married Clients

In addition to all of the above:

1. Increase MMMNA of CS
2. Increase CSRA
3. Increase countable assets prior to snapshot (50% states)

   a) Reverse mortgage
   b) Home equity loan
   c) Borrow from children

d) House into revocable trust

4. Spousal refusal ("just say no")
5. Transfer to trust for sole benefit of spouse
6. Divorce

Avoiding Estate Recovery

1. Change title to avoid probate (in probate-only state)

    a) Ladybird deed
    b) Small percentage gift of real estate w right of survivorship
    c) Revocable trust funding
    d) Title auto JTWROS (joint w right of survivorship)

2. Transfer home just before death

3. Gift house 5 yrs in advance

    a) outright to children, retaining life estate
    b) outright to trust, retaining life estate
    c) outright to trust, w occupancy agreement

4. Sell house

    a) move in with child and buy life estate or % interest

5. Buy new house jointly w child w right of survivorship

6. If disabled child:

    a) gift house to child or trust f/b/o child

        i. sign occupancy agreement

    b) gift remainder interest to child or trust f/b/o child

7. Avoid or minimize elective share

    a) Elective share amount in trust within CS's will
    b) Special Needs Trust of balance within CS's will, or to children

INDEX